DATE DUE

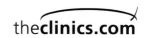
theclinics.com

Agnes E. Rupley, DVM, Dipl. ABVP–Avian
CONSULTING EDITOR

VETERINARY CLINICS

OF NORTH AMERICA

Exotic Animal Practice

Neuroanatomy and Neurodiagnostics

GUEST EDITORS
Lisa A. Tell, DVM, Dipl. ABVP–Avian
Marguerite F. Knipe, DVM, Dipl. ACVIM
(Neurology)

September 2007 • Volume 10 • Number 3

SAUNDERS
An Imprint of Elsevier, Inc.
PHILADELPHIA   LONDON   TORONTO   MONTREAL   SYDNEY   TOKYO

W.B. SAUNDERS COMPANY
A Division of Elsevier Inc.

Elsevier, Inc., 1600 John F. Kennedy Blvd., Suite 1800, Philadelphia, PA 19103-2899

http://www.vetexotic.theclinics.com

VETERINARY CLINICS OF NORTH AMERICA:	Volume 10, Number 3
EXOTIC ANIMAL PRACTICE	ISSN 1094-9194
September 2007	ISBN-13: 978-1-4160-5135-0
Editor: John Vassallo; j.vassallo@elsevier.com	ISBN-10: 1-4160-5135-X

Veterinary Clinics of North America: Exotic Animal Practice (ISSN 1094-9194) is published in January, May, and September by Elsevier, Inc.; Business and Editorial offices: 1600 John F. Kennedy Blvd., Suite 1800, Philadelphia, PA 19103-2899. Customer Service Office: 6277 Sea Harbor Drive, Orlando, FL 32887-4800. Subscription prices are $146.00 per year for US individuals, $253.00 per year for US institutions, $76.00 per year for US students and residents, $173.00 per year for Canadian individuals, $292.00 per year for Canadian institutions, $184.00 per year for international individuals, $292.00 per year for international institutions and $92.00 per year for Canadian and foreign students/residents. To receive student/resident rate, orders must be accompanied by name of affiliated institution, date of term, and the *signature* of program/residency coordinator on institution letterhead. Orders will be billed at individual rate until proof of status is received. Foreign air speed delivery is included in all *Clinics* subscription prices. All prices are subject to change without notice.

POSTMASTER: Send address changes to *Veterinary Clinics of North America: Exotic Animal Practice*; Elsevier Periodicals Customer Service, 6277 Sea Harbor Drive, Orlando, FL 32887-4800. **Customer Service: 1-800-654-2452 (US). From outside of the US, call 1-407-345-1000.**

Veterinary Clinics of North America: Exotic Animal Practice is covered in *Index Medicus.*

Printed in the United States of America.

CONSULTING EDITOR

AGNES E. RUPLEY, DVM, Diplomate, American Board of Veterinary Practitioners–Avian; Director and Chief Veterinarian, All Pets Medical & Laser Surgical Center, College Station, Texas

GUEST EDITORS

LISA A. TELL, DVM, Diplomate, American Board of Veterinary Practitioners–Avian; Professor, Department of Medicine and Epidemiology, School of Veterinary Medicine, University of California–Davis, Davis, California

MARGUERITE F. KNIPE, DVM, Diplomate, American College of Veterinary Internal Medicine (Neurology); Staff Veterinarian, Department of Surgical and Radiological Sciences, School of Veterinary Medicine, University of California–Davis, Davis, California

CONTRIBUTORS

R. AVERY BENNETT, DVM, MS, Diplomate, American College of Veterinary Surgeons; Professor of Soft Tissue Surgery, Department of Veterinary Clinical Medicine, College of Veterinary Medicine, University of Illinois, Urbana, Illinois

G.A. BRADSHAW, PhD, Director, The Kerulos Centre for Animal Psychology and Trauma Recovery, Environmental Science Graduate Program, Oregon State University, Corvallis, Oregon; and Pacifica Graduate Institute, Carpinteria, California

TRACY L. CLIPPINGER, DVM, Diplomate, American College of Zoological Medicine; Senior Veterinarian, Department of Veterinary Services, Zoological Society of San Diego-San Diego Zoo, San Diego, California

ORLANDO DIAZ-FIGUEROA, DVM, MS, Diplomate, American Board of Veterinary Practitioners–Avian Practice; Lake Howell Animal Clinic, Maitland, Florida

MARGUERITE F. KNIPE, DVM, Diplomate, American College of Veterinary Internal Medicine (Neurology); Staff Veterinarian, Department of Surgical and Radiological Sciences, School of Veterinary Medicine, University of California–Davis, Davis, California

RICHARD A. LECOUTEUR, BVSc, PhD, Diplomate, American College of Veterinary Internal Medicine (Neurology); Professor of Neurology/Neurosurgery, Department of Surgical and Radiological Sciences, School of Veterinary Medicine, University of California–Davis, Davis, California

CHRISTOPHER L. MARIANI, DVM, PhD, Assistant Professor of Neurology and Neurosurgery, Department of Clinical Sciences, College of Veterinary Medicine, North Carolina State University, Raleigh, North Carolina

SUSAN E. OROSZ, PhD, Diplomate, American Board of Veterinary Practitioners (Avian); Diplomate, European College of Avian Medicine and Surgery; Bird and Exotic Pet Wellness Center, Toledo, Ohio

ANNA OSOFSKY, DVM, Diplomate, American Board of Veterinary Practitioners–Avian Practice; Associate Veterinarian, Carrollton West Pet Hospital, Carrollton, Texas

SIMON R. PLATT, BVMS, MCRVS, Diplomate, American College of Veterinary Internal Medicine; Diplomate, European College of Veterinary Neurology; Associate Professor, Department of Small Animal Medicine and Surgery, College of Veterinary Medicine, University of Georgia, Athens, Georgia

MARY O. SMITH, BVM&S, PhD, Diplomate, American College of Veterinary Internal Medicine (Neurology); Affiliated Veterinary Specialists, Maitland, Florida

KAREN M. VERNAU, DVM, MAS, Diplomate, American College of Veterinary Internal Medicine (Neurology); Assistant Professor of Clinical Neurology/Neurosurgery, Department of Surgical and Radiological Sciences, School of Veterinary Medicine, University of California–Davis, Davis, California

SETH WALLACK, DVM, Diplomate, American College of Veterinary Radiologists; Veterinary Imaging Center of San Diego, Inc. and DVMinsight-premier teleradiology, San Diego, California

JEANETTE WYNEKEN, PhD, Associate Professor of Biological Sciences, Department of Biological Sciences, Florida Atlantic University, Boca Raton, Florida

CONTENTS

use available diagnostic tests to confirm the presence of neurologic diseases. Recent advances in ferret medicine and veterinary neurology offer new capabilities to investigate and treat neurological disease in ferrets.

Several significant advances in understanding brain-behavior development have made a critical contribution to clinical assessment of companion birds. First, psychobiological health and its dysfunctions now are understood as the product of nature and nurture and therefore exquisitely sensitive to stressors effected by altered socio-ecological conditions within and across generations. Second, discoveries associated with avian brain evolution and ethology show that emotional and cognitive capacities of birds are comparable to mammals. This article presents an overview of these new perspectives and, following, discusses specific, clinically relevant anatomy of the avian central nervous system. By understanding the location of these tracts and their function and the location of the cranial nerves and their nuclei in the brain stem, the clinician can understand and perform the neurological examination, better interpret findings, and localize lesions.

The purpose of this article is to guide the avian clinician in the assessment of neurologic function in birds. Physical and neurologic examinations that evaluate cranial nerves, postural reactions, and spinal reflexes identify neurologic dysfunction and the corresponding anatomic location of the lesion. Ancillary diagnostic tests, such as cerebrospinal fluid analysis, diagnostic imaging, muscle and nerve histology, and electrodiagnostics, are tools to confirm and clarify conclusions from the neurologic examination and to identify the cause of disease. Once the disease location and pathologic process have been identified, appropriate treatment and prognosis may be provided.

The reptilian nervous system is relatively simple in structure yet is characterized by great functional diversity. This article describes the reptilian nervous system, highlighting the similarities and differences among species in structures and functions.

FORTHCOMING ISSUES

RECENT ISSUES

ELSEVIER
SAUNDERS

VETERINARY
CLINICS
Exotic Animal Practice

Vet Clin Exot Anim 10 (2007) ix

Preface

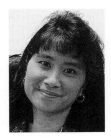 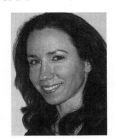

Lisa A. Tell,
DVM, DABVP–Avian

Marguerite F. Knipe,
DVM, DACVIM (Neurology)

Guest Editors

Veterinarians who practice avian, reptile, and exotic small animal medicine are faced with increasingly complex cases that encompass multiple organ systems. The neurologic system and diseases associated with it present challenges to practitioners, especially in species that are less tractable. In this issue of *Veterinary Clinics of North America: Exotic Animal Practice*, numerous distinguished worldwide experts in neurology and avian, reptile, and exotic small animal medicine have combined their efforts to provide insight and knowledge regarding the unique anatomy of birds, reptiles, and exotic small mammals and neurodiagnostic procedures that can be used for these patients. These articles highlight the unique anatomic characteristics of the species, the diseases that should be present on the differential list, and the diagnostic tests that might be used for gaining a diagnosis. This issue is meant to provide specialized information for dedicated practitioners who are always willing to seek new knowledge and strategies that will help advance the profession of exotic animal medicine and contribute to the needs of their patients and human guardians.

Lisa A. Tell, DVM, DABVP–Avian
Marguerite F. Knipe, DVM, DACVIM (Neurology)
School of Veterinary Medicine
University of California–Davis, Davis, CA, USA

E-mail addresses: latell@ucdavis.edu
mfknipe@ucdavis.edu

1094-9194/07/$ - see front matter © 2007 Elsevier Inc. All rights reserved.
doi:10.1016/j.cvex.2007.05.002

ELSEVIER
SAUNDERS

VETERINARY
CLINICS
Exotic Animal Practice

Vet Clin Exot Anim 10 (2007) 713–730

Functional Neuroanatomy of the Domestic Rabbit (*Oryctolagus cuniculus*)

Anna Osofsky, DVM, DABVP-Avian Practice[a],
Richard A. LeCouteur, BVSc, PhD, DACVIM
(Neurology)[b], Karen M. Vernau, DVM, MAS,
DACVIM (Neurology)[b],*

[a]*Carrollton West Pet Hospital, Carrollton, TX 75007, USA*
[b]*Department of Surgical and Radiological Sciences, School of Veterinary Medicine, University of California–Davis, Davis, CA 95616, USA*

This article provides a clinically relevant review of the neuroanatomy of the central nervous system of the domestic rabbit (*Oryctolagus cuniculus*) that will help guide veterinarians in localizing neurological disease in this species. The vertebral column, spinal cord and brain of rabbits are similar to those of other mammals; however, where they exist, features unique to the rabbit are emphasized.

The vertebral column

In most domestic rabbits, the vertebral column is composed of seven cervical, 12 thoracic, seven lumbar, four sacral, and 15 to 16 caudal vertebrae [1–3]. Some individual variation occurs; there are reports of rabbits with 13 thoracic vertebrae and six lumbar vertebrae [4,5]. In one study that evaluated 64 New Zealand white rabbits, 43.8% had 12 thoracic and seven lumbar vertebrae; 32.8% had 13 thoracic and six lumbar vertebrae, and 23.4% had 13 thoracic and seven lumbar vertebrae [5]. As in other mammals, the first two cervical vertebrae are specialized, forming the atlas and the axis. The atlas articulates directly with the occipital region of the skull. The axis incorporates the cranial projecting odontoid process, which allows the atlas to rotate on the axis [1]. The lumbar vertebrae of rabbits have several differences from other domestic mammals (Fig. 1). The first three lumbar vertebrae have a ventral crest. The ventral

---

* Corresponding author.
E-mail address: kmvernau@ucdavis.edu (K.M. Vernau).

doi:10.1016/j.cvex.2007.04.007   *vetexotic.theclinics.com*

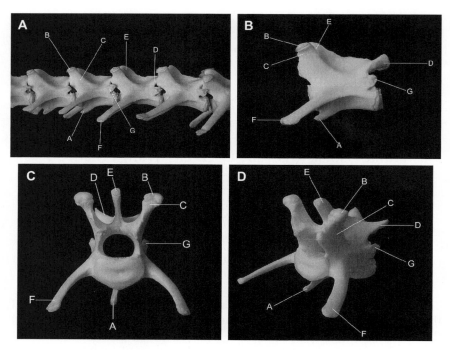

Fig. 1. (*A*) Domestic rabbit (*Oryctolagus cuniculus*) lumbar vertebral skeleton (left lateral view). (*B*) Left lateral view of second lumbar vertebra. (*C*) Second lumbar vertebra (cranial surface). (*D*) Second lumbar vertebra (lateral oblique view).
A - Ventral crest. B - Mammillary process of cranial articular process. C - Cranial articular process. D - Caudal articular process. E - Spinous process. F - Transverse process. G - Accessory process.

crest may be very large in some species of wild rabbits (Fig. 2). All lumbar vertebrae have a prominent mammillary process of the cranial articular process, where the powerful lumbar musculature attaches to the vertebral column [1]. Unlike other domestic mammals, the dorsal aspect of the lumbar vertebral mammillary process is level with, or slightly ventral to, the spinous process. The first three vertebrae of the sacrum are fused, while the fourth sacral vertebra is fused variably [1].

The spinal cord

The rabbit spinal cord is similar to that of other mammals (Fig. 3). It is enclosed by the meninges (dura mater, arachnoid and pia mater). The dura mater is the outermost layer, and the pia mater the innermost layer. The dura mater is a thick, fibrous layer. The arachnoid mater is a very thin membrane, continuous with the dura mater. Fine connective tissue filaments that resemble a spider web extend from the arachnoid mater to the pia mater.

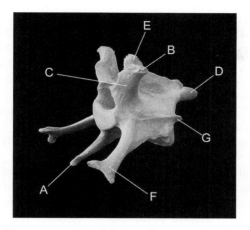

Fig. 2. Wild rabbit (Eastern cottontail; *Sylvilagus floridanus*), first lumbar vertebra (oblique view). Note the flared distal end of the transverse process F and the large ventral crest A. B - Mammillary process of cranial articular process. C - Cranial articular process. D - Caudal articular process. E - Spinous process. G - Accessory process.

The space that lies between the arachnoid and the pia mater is the subarachnoid space, which contains cerebrospinal fluid (CSF) [6].

In the center of the spinal cord is the small central canal, lined by a thin layer of ependymal cells (Fig. 3). It contains CSF and is continuous with the ventricular system of the brain. The spinal cord is composed of gray and white matter. The gray matter is in the center of the spinal cord and is butterfly- or H-shaped in transverse section, and the white matter is peripheral to the gray matter [2,7]. The gray matter contains nerve cell bodies and unmyelinated or thinly myelinated axons, and it is divided into three horns: the ventral, dorsal, and intermediolateral horns. The ventral horn contains

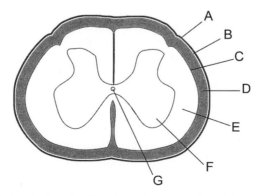

Fig. 3. Diagram of the spinal cord and meninges (transverse view). (*A*) Dura mater. (*B*) Arachnoid mater. (*C*) Pia mater. (*D*) Subarachnoid space (with cerebrospinal fluid). (*E*) White matter. (*F*) Gray matter. (*G*) Central canal.

mostly motor nerve cell bodies, and the dorsal horn contains the cell bodies of interneurons. The sensory nerve cell bodies lie in the dorsal root ganglia, outside of the spinal cord. The intermediolateral horn is located between the ventral and dorsal horns and is the smallest of the three. It contains the cell bodies of the preganglionic sympathetic neurons in the thoracolumbar region, and preganglionic parasympathetic neurons in the sacral region of the spinal cord [6,7]. The white matter consists of myelinated axons forming ascending and descending tracts [6,7].

At birth, the spinal cord of the rabbit extends the length of the vertebral canal. After birth, the spinal cord and vertebral column have differential growth rates, and as a result, at maturity, the spinal cord is shorter than the vertebral column. Therefore, spinal cord segments and nerve roots are not necessarily housed within vertebrae of the same number (Fig. 4) [2]. The disproportionate growth of the spinal cord relative to the vertebral canal causes the caudal spinal nerves to develop more cranially than the point at which they exit the vertebral column, leading to formation of the cauda equina [2]. The cauda equina is less pronounced compared with people, because the spinal cord extends more caudally in the rabbit (Fig. 4) [2].

The spinal cord arises at the foramen magnum and extends almost the length of the vertebral canal; it may terminate within the first, second, or third sacral vertebra, but most commonly within the second sacral vertebra [5]. In rabbits with a greater number of vertebrae (eg, 13 thoracic and seven lumbar vertebrae), the spinal cord terminates more cranially than in rabbits with 12 thoracic vertebrae [2,5]. The number of paired spinal nerve roots parallels the number of vertebrae (except in the cervical region where there are seven cervical vertebrae and eight spinal nerves). The first cervical spinal nerve emerges through the lateral vertebral foramen of the atlas. The remainder of the cervical spinal nerves are numbered according to the vertebra lying caudal to the intervertebral foramina they exit. Spinal nerve C8 exits the C7-T1 intervertebral foramen, and the remainder of the spinal nerves are numbered according to the vertebra lying cranial to the intervertebral foramina [2]. Thus, most rabbits have eight cervical, 12 thoracic, seven lumbar, and four sacral pairs of spinal nerves [2,5,8]. Rabbits have 15 or 16 caudal vertebrae, and therefore are likely to have 15 or 16 pairs of caudal nerve roots, despite reference in the literature to only six caudal pairs of caudal nerve roots [2].

Each spinal cord segment has a ventral and a dorsal nerve root within the vertebral canal on each side. Each nerve root consists of numerous rootlets at the level of the spinal cord. The dorsal rootlets contain afferent fibers entering the spinal cord at the dorsolateral sulcus. The ventral rootlets contain efferent fibers that are exiting the spinal cord at the ventrolateral sulcus. The dorsal nerve root has a dorsal root ganglion that contains nerve cell bodies. The dorsal and the ventral roots combine to form the spinal nerve at the level of the intervertebral foramen. Distal to the intervertebral foramen, the spinal nerve divides into a dorsal, ventral, and visceral (communicating)

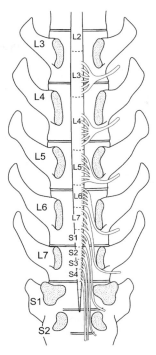

Fig. 4. Lumbar spinal cord and nerve roots (dorsal lamina removed) of a New Zealand White domestic rabbit (*Oryctolagus cuniculus*). Note the relationship of the lumbosacral spinal cord segments and the vertebral bodies in a rabbit with 12 thoracic vertebrae and seven lumbar vertebrae. The spinal cord terminates at the S2 vertebral body. (*Modified from* Greenaway J, Partlow G, Gonsholt N, et al. Anatomy of the lumbosacral spinal cord in rabbits. J Am Anim Hosp Assoc 2001;37:27–34.)

ramus [2,9]. The ventral branches are the most important clinically, because they continue as the peripheral nerves that innervate the limb musculature.

There are two enlargements of the spinal cord: the brachial and lumbar enlargements or intumescences [7]. These spinal cord regions are enlarged, because they contain an increased number of neurons and cell bodies whose axons innervate the muscles of the thoracic and pelvic limbs [6]. The brachial enlargement is located in the caudal cervical region and contains cervical 5, 6, 7, 8, and thoracic 1 (C5-T1) spinal cord segments [7]. The brachial plexus is formed by the ventral rami of the cervical spinal nerves C5-T1 that innervate the musculature of the thoracic limb. The lumbar enlargement of the spinal cord comprises spinal cord segments lumbar (L) 4, 5, 6, 7, and sacral (S) 1, 2, 3, 4, and the caudal (Cd) segments (Figs. 4 and 5). The spinal nerves from L4-Cd form the lumbosacral plexus once they exit the vertebral canal to innervate the musculature of the pelvic limb, bladder, anus, and perineum [7].

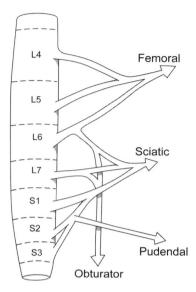

Fig. 5. Lumbosacral nerve root contributions to the nerves of the pelvic limb and perineum of a New Zealand White domestic rabbit (*Oryctolagus cuniculus*). Note the typical nerve root contributions in a rabbit with 12 thoracic vertebrae and seven lumbar vertebrae (*Modified from* Greenaway J, Partlow G, Gonsholt N, et al. Anatomy of the lumbosacral spinal cord in rabbits. J Am Anim Hosp Assoc 2001;37:27–34.)

The spinal nerves of the lumbar enlargement originate in an anatomically similar location in the rabbit as the cat and horse, as the spinal cord terminates within the sacral region in all three species [5]. In one study, the spinal cord of New Zealand white rabbits terminated at S2 in almost 80% of the animals [5]. In the study of New Zealand white rabbits, in those with 12 thoracic and seven lumbar vertebrae, the femoral nerve was formed by contributions from nerve roots L4 through L6, the obturator nerve by nerve roots L6 and L7, the sciatic nerve by L6, L7, S1, and S2, and the pudendal nerve by nerve roots S2 and S3 [5]. In contrast, pelvic limb muscles of rabbits with 13 thoracic and six lumbar vertebrae had the following nerve root origins: nerve roots L3 to 5 contributed to the femoral nerve and the obturator nerve; nerve roots L5, L6, S1, S2, and S3 contributed to the sciatic nerve, and nerve roots S2 and S3 contributed to the pudendal nerve [5].

The autonomic nervous system consists of the thoracolumbar or sympathetic division and the craniosacral or parasympathetic division. The sympathetic division consists of nerve fibers in the tectotegmental pathway that run in the intermediolateral part of the gray matter, and two longitudinal trunks that run laterally ventral to the vertebral column [3]. These sympathetic trunks are formed from fibers extending from the ventral roots of the spinal nerves by means of communicating rami [3]. There is a sympathetic ganglion at each junction with a communicating ramus [3]. There also are sympathetic ganglia separate from the sympathetic chains that are important in visceral function. These separate ganglia consist of the cranial and caudal cervical ganglia and the lumbar-located celiac ganglion and its associated celiac plexus [3]. The parasympathetic division's preganglionic axons exit the brain as part of cranial nerves (CN) III, VII, IX, and X and exit the sacrum with the ventral roots of the sacral nerves [9].

Spinal cord pathways

Rabbits use various gaits when moving slowly, but most hop at high speeds [10]. Hopping is thought to give rabbits an energetic advantage over nonhopping quadripedal mammals, especially at high hopping speeds. Neuronal networks in the spinal cord are capable of producing rhythmic movements, including walking and hopping. These spinal networks are referred to as central pattern generators or CPGs [11]. Experiments using domestic rabbits showed that an intact lumbosacral spinal cord and cranial two thirds of the pons are required for hopping [12]. Specific information regarding CPGs of the rabbit spinal cord, and the role of CPGs in generating hopping movements, however, is lacking.

Clinicians must be aware that, similar to cats and dogs, a rabbit with a severed spinal cord may move the pelvic limbs under certain conditions. Experiments using domestic rabbits with spinal cords transected at the last thoracic vertebral level (spinal rabbits) were capable of alternating movements of the pelvic limbs, when the pelvic limb toes touched the ground [10]. When the apparatus supporting the rabbits was moved forward slowly, a synchronous movement of the pelvic limbs (hop) was observed [10].

Despite the differences noted regarding limb movements, the rabbit has been used widely as an animal model in human spinal cord research. Little information, however, is available regarding the importance and relative size of spinal cord tracts in this species. As rabbits most likely have similar spinal cord pathways to other domestic mammals, only the most important pathways are discussed in the following section.

Ascending pathways

Dorsal column medial lemniscus pathway

This pathway contains large myelinated axons that carry the sensory modalities of mechanoreception (from the thoracic and pelvic limbs) and conscious proprioception from the thoracic limbs. Primary neurons enter the spinal cord from the periphery and travel ipsilaterally in the fasciculus gracilis (caudal to T6) and the fasciculus cuneatus (cranial to T6) to the nucleus gracilis and cuneatus in the medulla (caudal to the fourth ventricle), where they synapse. Second-order neurons then decussate (cross the midline) to travel by means of the medial lemniscus to synapse in the thalamus.

Third-order neurons travel from the thalamus to the ipsilateral cerebral cortex by means of the internal capsule [6].

Spinomedullothalamic pathways

This pathway is important for unconscious and conscious proprioception from the pelvic limbs. First-order neurons enter the spinal cord and travel in the fasciculus gracilis. Second-order neurons travel cranially in the dorsolateral funiculus of the spinal cord to the nucleus Z in the medulla. Third-order neurons exit this nucleus and decussate to ascend in the medial lemniscus to the thalamus, where they synapse. Fourth-order neurons then travel to the ipsilateral cerebral cortex by means of the internal capsule [6].

Descending pathways

Corticospinal tract

The primary efferent pathways from the motor cortex (cerebrum) of people are termed pyramidal tracts. In people, pyramidal tracts include the corticospinal tract and the corticobulbar tract. The corticospinal tract travels from the motor cortex to the contralateral spinal cord and is involved in fine voluntary movements of the limbs. The corticobulbar pathways travel from the motor cortex to the contralateral nuclei of cranial nerves that are involved in fine movements of the muscles of the head. In rabbits, the corticobulbar pathway is well-developed, reflecting the fine movements seen in the head muscles of rabbits. The corticospinal tract in rabbits extends only to the cervical level, however, reflecting the relative lack of fine voluntary movements seen in the limbs of rabbits when compared with people [13].

Rubrospinal tract

The rubrospinal tract is the primary pathway involved in locomotion and posture of quadripeds. This tract originates in the motor cortex, before synapsing in the red nucleus of the midbrain, immediately decussating within the midbrain, and then descending in the spinal cord in the lateral funiculus before projecting (predominantly) to gamma lower motor neurons [6].

Vestibulospinal tracts

There are two vestibulospinal tracts (lateral and medial). The lateral vestibulospinal tract arises from the lateral vestibular nucleus and descends the length of the spinal cord in the ventral funiculus without decussating. It projects to the alpha motor neurons, and it is strongly facilitatory to extensor muscles, and inhibitory to flexor muscles of the limbs. The medial vestibulospinal tract arises from the medial vestibular nucleus and descends in the ipsilateral spinal cord in the dorsal part of the ventral funiculus, to the cranial thoracic spinal cord. The fibers in the medial vestibulospinal tract are important for maintaining head position [6].

The skull

The bones of the rabbit skull are similar to those of dogs, but the rabbit has many bones with a spongy texture containing wide medullary cavities, compared with the smooth, hard skull of the dog (Figs. 6 and 7) [1,4]. Rabbit tympanic bullae are much larger than those of dogs, and the external auditory meatus is longer and more tubular in shape [1]. The zygomatic arch of the rabbit is much flatter than in the dog, causing rabbits to have a narrow skull [1] that may permit rabbits to burrow more easily. The laterally placed eyes allow for a visual field that is almost a complete sphere (Fig. 8) [4,14]. The foramina of the rabbit skull are likely to be similar to those of the dog, although precise nomenclature in the rabbit apparently is lacking [1,3].

Brain

An understanding of functional anatomy of the rabbit brain is essential for clinicians to accurately localize a problem to the correct area of the central nervous system. The brain of the rabbit is organized anatomically as in other mammals [2]. It is enveloped in the meninges, consisting of the outer dura mater, the arachnoid, and the inner pia mater [7]. The dura mater is adherent to the periosteum of the skull. Embryologically, the dura originates as two layers, and in some regions, it splits into a periosteal layer and an

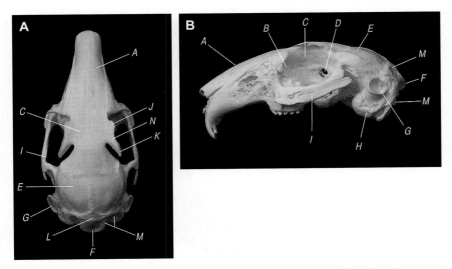

Fig. 6. Lateral (*A*) and dorsal (*B*) views of the skull of the domestic rabbit (*Oryctolagus cuniculus*).
A - Nasal bone. B - Lacrimal bone. C - Frontal bone. D - Optic foramen. E - Parietal bone. F - External occipital protuberance. G - External auditory meatus. H - Tympanic bulla. I - Zygomatic bone. J - Cranial supraorbital process of the frontal bone. K - Caudal supraorbital process of the frontal bone. L - Interparietal bone. M - Occipital bone. N - Zygomatic process of the frontal bone.

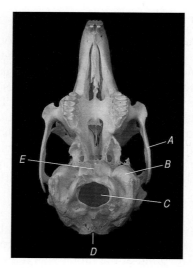

Fig. 7. Ventral view of the skull of the domestic rabbit (*Oryctolagus cuniculus*).
A - Zygomatic bone. B - Tympanic bulla. C - Foramen magnum. D - External occipital protuberance. E - Basisphenoid bone.

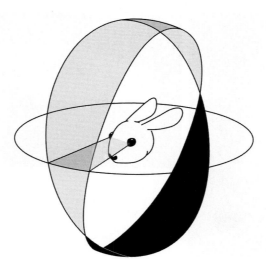

Fig. 8. Topography of the visual field in the domestic rabbit (*Oryctolagus cuniculus*). Note the small area of binocular vision in the horizontal plane, about 30 degrees. Binocular vision is denoted by the gray shaded area and the blind sector by the black shaded area. Monocular vision is denoted by the white areas contained within the sphere. Note the position of the blind sector, ventral and behind the head. (*Modified from* Hughes A. Topographical relationships between the anatomy and physiology of the rabbit visual system. Documenta Ophthalmologica 1971;30: 30–159.)

inner layer. The inner layer of the dura mater forms partitions between parts of the brain, including the falx cerebri between the cerebral hemispheres, and the tentorium cerebelli between the cerebellum and cerebrum [4,8].

The forebrain consists of the telencephalon and diencephalon. The telencephalon comprises the cerebrum (cerebral cortices and basal nuclei), the largest single structure of the brain [7]. In contrast to dogs, the rabbit's cerebral cortex is lissencephalic, or smooth, because of the lack of gyri (Figs. 9 and 10) [13]. The most rostral portions of the brain are the ventrally located olfactory bulbs [7]. The cerebral hemispheres are divided longitudinally by the sagittal fissure; the ventral border of the fissure is formed by the corpus callosum, which is a white matter tract connecting the two cerebral hemispheres [4,8].

The diencephalon is located ventral to the telencephalon and consists of the metathalamus, thalamus, hypothalamus, pineal gland (epithalamus), and the pituitary gland. The optic chiasm also is located in the diencephalon [7]. Except for the sense of olfaction, all sensory pathways must travel through the thalamus to reach the cerebral cortex [15]. The medial and lateral geniculate nuclei form the metathalamus; the former is an important part of the auditory pathway, while the latter is part of the visual pathway [9].

The midbrain (mesencephalon) is located caudal to the diencephalon and consists of the dorsal tectum (Latin = roof) and ventral tegmentum (Latin = covering). The tectum comprises the rostral and caudal colliculi, involved with visual and auditory reflexes, respectively. The rostral colliculi are larger

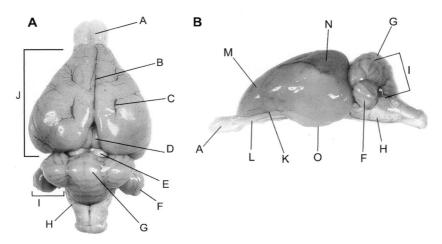

Fig. 9. Dorsal (*A*) and lateral (*B*) views of the unpreserved brain of a New Zealand White domestic rabbit (*Oryctolagus cuniculus*).
A - Olfactory bulb. B - Longitudinal fissure. C - Marginal sulcus. D - Rostral colliculus. E - Caudal colliculus. F - Cerebellar paraflocculus. G - Cerebellar vermis. H - Medulla. I - Cerebellar hemisphere. J - Cerebral cortex. K- Lateral rhinal sulcus. L - Olfactory peduncle. M - Frontal lobe of cerebrum. N - Occipital lobe of cerebrum. O - Pyriform lobe of cerebrum.

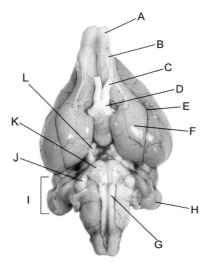

Fig. 10. Ventral view of the unpreserved brain of a New Zealand White domestic rabbit
(*Oryctolagus cuniculus*).
A - Olfactory bulb. B - Olfactory peduncle. C - Optic nerve (CN II). D - Optic chiasm. E - Lateral rhinal sulcus. F - Pyriform lobe of cerebrum. G - Pyramids. H - Cerebellar paraflocculus. I - Cerebellar hemisphere. J - Trigeminal nerve. K - Pons. L - Oculomotor nerve (CN III).

than the caudal colliculi in rabbits (Fig. 9A) [2]. Unlike dogs and cats, the rostral and caudal colliculi of rabbits are clearly visible when the dorsal aspect of the brain is examined. Important structures in the tegmentum are the mesencephalic aqueduct, the red nucleus, and the reticular formation (reticular activating system) [7]. The motor nucleus of CN III (oculomotor nerve) is located close to the midline, just ventral to the peri-aqueductal gray matter that surrounds the mesencephalic aqueduct. It is located more cranial than the motor nucleus of CN IV (trochlear nerve). CN III emerges from the ventro–medial aspect of the cerebral peduncle. The oculomotor nerve innervates most of the extrinsic muscles of the eye, the upper eyelid, and the pupil. The nucleus of CN IV is close to the midline, ventral to the peri-aqueductal gray matter. Axons from the CN IV nucleus exit the midbrain dorsally, in the rostral medullary velum, just rostral to the cerebellar peduncles. The trochlear nerve then decussates, to innervate the contralateral dorsal oblique muscle of the eye [4].

The hindbrain or rhombencephalon consists of the cerebellum, pons, and medulla; the cerebellum and pons form the metencephalon, while the medulla forms the caudal-most part of the brain, the myelencephalon [7]. The thalamus, hypothalamus, midbrain, pons, and medulla together constitute the brainstem [7]. Diseases such encephalitozoonosis and central extension of otitis media–interna affect the brainstem in rabbits [16]. Cranial nerves V to XII arise in the hindbrain.

As in other mammals, the cerebellum consists of the central vermis and the laterally located right and left cerebellar hemispheres [7]. Rabbits have prominent paraflocculi, which are ventrolateral extensions of the cerebellar hemispheres (Figs. 9 and 10) [4]. The paraflocculus remains entirely separate from the flocculus at all stages of embryonic development, but it maintains connections with the pyramis and uvula. These structures are part of the paleocerebellum, phylogenetically the second oldest part of the cerebellum [17]. The flocculus has been studied extensively in rabbits because of its importance in the adaptation of the vestibulocular reflex, and in sensory and sensorimotor integration for retinal image stabilization [18]. Although the precise functions of the large parafloculi of rabbits remain incompletely understood, it is likely that they have significance with regard to vestibular functions and eye movements. In the midsagittal plane, the cerebellum has a triangular shape, rather than the more round shape seen in other domestic animals (eg, dog, cat, horse, sheep).

The pons is located just caudal to the cerebral peduncles. The ventral part of the pons contains the transverse pontine fibers that extend transversely across the ventral aspect of the brain into the cerebellar peduncles. The dorsal part of the pons contains the nuclei for CN V (trigeminal nerve). The medulla oblongata connects the brain with the spinal cord; the rostral medulla contains the nuclei of CN VI (abducens nerve), CN VII (facial nerve), CN VIII (vestibulocochlear nerve), the pyramids, and the trapezoid body [2]. The pyramids of the medulla are ventrally located narrow tracts that extend from just caudal to the pons to the level of the spinomedullary junction. The pyramids are axons in the corticospinal tract, which originate from cell bodies in the cerebral cortex and terminate in the cervical region of the spinal cord (see Fig. 10) [4,9]. In rodents, however, the corticospinal tracts terminate in the sacral segments of the spinal cord [19]. The trapezoid body of the medulla also is located ventrally [4], but is dorsal and lateral to the pyramids, and consists of transverse fibers that extend from the ventral cochlear nucleus. The mid- to caudal medulla consists of the olivary nucleus, the lateral cuneate nucleus, the reticular formation, and the nuclei of CN IX to XII (glossopharyngeal, vagus, accessory, and hypoglossal nerves). The reticular formation is a diffuse network of nerve cell bodies and fibers that is important for maintaining arousal.

The ventricles and choroid plexi of the rabbit are arranged similarly to other mammals. Unlike dogs, cats and sheep, however, rabbits have a funnel-shaped mesencephalic aqueduct, with the widest diameter being rostral [2].

The cranial nerves

An understanding of the anatomy and function of the cranial nerves is essential in order for the clinician to localize the lesion in the nervous system of a rabbit.

Olfactory nerve

The olfactory nerve is responsible for the sense of smell [2]. The cell body of the olfactory nerve (neuron 1) is in the olfactory epithelium [9]. The axon of neuron 1 passes through the multiple small foramina in the cribriform plate of the skull, to the olfactory bulb where it synapses with neuron 2. Rabbits have a relatively large olfactory bulb located at the rostral aspect of each cerebral hemisphere (Figs. 9 and 10) [2,7]. The axon of neuron 2 travels caudally in the olfactory peduncle, where it divides into the lateral and medial olfactory tracts. The axons in the lateral olfactory tract synapse with neuron 3 in the ipsilateral olfactory tubercle; some axons in the medial olfactory tract decussate and synapse with neuron 3 in the contralateral olfactory tubercle. The axon of neuron 3 travels from its cell body in the olfactory tubercle to the pyriform lobe. As previously stated, this is the only sensory pathway that does not involve the thalamus [6].

Optic nerve

The rabbit visual field forms an almost compete sphere [14]. In the horizontal plane, rabbits have about 30 degrees of binocular vision, which extends to about 70 degrees beyond vertical above their head. In front of their head, the field of binocular vision extends 30 to 40 degrees below horizontal. Therefore, they do not have binocular vision behind their head in the horizontal plane. Rabbits have a narrow blind sector under and behind their heads, (Fig. 8) [14], which is interesting, as it is not in a position from which a predator might be expected to approach.

The optic nerve is the afferent (sensory) pathway for vision. Neuron 1 is the retinal bipolar cell, and neuron 2 is the retinal ganglion cell [7,9]. The axons of neuron 2 form the optic nerve. The optic nerve is covered by meninges and travels through the optic foramen in the skull to reach the optic chiasm. Most of the optic nerve fibers in the rabbit decussate at the optic chiasm, as is generally the case in mammals with laterally located eyes and, thus, panoramic visual fields [2,13]. The optic tract travels from the ventrally located optic chiasm to the lateral geniculate body and the rostral colliculus [2]. The lateral geniculate body acts as a relay of visual information to the cerebral cortex for conscious visual experience [2]. The rostral colliculus participates in reflex actions by sending information to the nuclei of cranial nerves involved with moving the eye (CN III, IV, and VI), the parasympathetic nucleus of CN III (to constrict their pupils), the reticular formation (to adjust the level of readiness), and the cervical spinal cord by means of the tectospinal pathway (to move the head and neck in response to visual stimuli [2,6].

Oculomotor nerve

The oculomotor nerve is the most important nerve for innervation of the muscles of the eye. This nerve contains motor fibers that innervate the extrinsic striated muscles of the eye and parasympathetic fibers that innervate the intrinsic ocular muscles [7]. The intrinsic muscles (ciliary and sphincter pupillae muscles) control the curvature of the lens and pupillary constriction/dilation respectively and are innervated by parasympathetic motor fibers from CN III. The extrinsic ocular striated muscles include the dorsal rectus, medial rectus, ventral rectus, and the ventral oblique muscles; these muscles are innervated by somatic efferent fibers. The oculo-motor nerve also innervates the levator palpebrae muscle of the dorsal eyelid. The somatic motor fibers of CN III originate in the midbrain, in the oculomotor nucleus [13]. The preganglionic fibers originate in the parasympathetic nucleus of CN III (also known as the Edinger-Westphal nucleus) located dorsal to the motor nucleus of CN III in the midbrain [13]. As in other species, CN III probably exits the skull through the orbital fissure (along with CN IV, the ophthalmic branch of CN V, and CN VI) [9] but to the authors' knowledge, this has not been reported.

Trochlear nerve

The trochlear nerve innervates the dorsal oblique muscle of the eye by means of somatic efferents from the trochlear nucleus. The trochlear nucleus is located in the roof of the midbrain [7], and contains approximately 900 neurons that mostly are motoneurons. The axons travel in the trochlear nerve and decussate in the rostral medullary velum to innervate the contra-lateral dorsal oblique muscle. Approximately 3% of trochlear motor neurons innervate the ipsilateral dorsal oblique muscle [20]. The tensor trochleae muscle is a muscle in the rabbit (not recognized in other mamma-lian species) innervated by approximately one third of the trochlear motor neurons. The function of this muscle is unknown [20]. The trochlear nerve is the only cranial nerve to emerge from the brainstem dorsally. Like other species, CN IV probably exits the skull through the orbital fissure [9], but to the authors' knowledge, this is not reported in the rabbit.

Trigeminal nerve

The trigeminal nerve consists of three branches: ophthalmic, maxillary, and mandibular. The ophthalmic and maxillary nerves are purely sensory, while the mandibular nerve is both sensory and motor. All three branches of CN V arise from the lateral portions of the pons [7]; there is a larger sensory root and a smaller motor root. The trigeminal nerve innervates the muscles of mastication [2]. The ophthalmic branch of CN V innervates the external eye and skin of the head, providing sensation to the face. The maxillary branch innervates the vibrissae and maxillary (upper) teeth. The mandibular branch provides motor innervation to the jaw and is sensory to the skin of the lower face, teeth of the mandible (lower jaw), mouth, and tongue [7]. These branches probably exit the skull as they do in other mammals. The ophthalmic branch exits the skull in the orbital fissure, the maxillary branch by means of the round foramen, and the mandibular branch through the oval foramen [9]. This has not been reported for the rabbit, however.

Abducens nerve

The abducens nerve innervates the lateral rectus and retractor bulbi muscles of the eye; thus, it controls lateral rotation of the eye and retraction of the globe [7,13,20]. It originates from the lateral aspect of the rostral part of the medulla [4,7]. CN VI probably exits the skull through the orbital fissure [9], but to the authors' knowledge, this has not been reported.

Facial nerve

The facial nerve is a mixed nerve. It is primarily a motor nerve to the muscles of the jaw and head (facial expression), but it also has a small sensory component to the palate and rostral two thirds of the tongue (taste) [1,2,7]. The facial nerve arises at the level of the trapezoid body of the medulla [7]. The facial nerve exits the cranial cavity by means of the internal acoustic meatus, where it travels in the facial canal. It exits the skull from the stylomastoid foramen that is just caudal to the external auditory meatus. The anatomy of the facial nerve varies fairly significantly between individuals [1]. Once it exits the skull, there is extensive branching of the nerve to supply the pinna, along with smaller branches to the angle of the jaw and areas caudal to the external auditory meatus [1]. The aforementioned major branch of the facial nerve (the dorsal buccal branch) extends from a point just ventral to the ear toward the nose; ventral to the eye this large branch divides into numerous smaller branches [1,21]. Ventral to the major branch, there are usually two smaller branches (the ventral buccal branch and the marginal mandibular branch) that extend to the ventral aspects of the masseter muscle, but there is much individual variation [1,21]. Like other mammals, the facial nerve most likely also innervates the lacrimal and salivary glands (parasympathetic).

Vestibulocochlear nerve

The vestibulocochlear nerve is associated closely with the facial nerve. The vestibulocochlear nerve is purely sensory, with the cochlear branch mediating hearing, and a vestibular branch mediating orientation of the head relative to gravity [2]. The auditory component of CN VIII terminates in the cochlear nucleus. Axons decussate after leaving the cochlear nucleus, forming the trapezoid body of the medulla. The axons then travel rostrally in the contralateral lateral lemniscus to the medial geniculate nucleus of the thalamus [2,7,15], and then through auditory radiation to the cerebral cortex.

Cell bodies of the vestibular division of CN VIII are in one of four vestibular nuclei in the medulla [15]. Because information about equilibrium is so essential for balance of the head and body, there are pathways from the vestibular nuclei to other locations in the brain stem, to the cerebellum, to the cerebral cortex, and to the spinal cord [15]. The vestibulocochlear nerve is the only cranial nerve that does not exit the skull.

Glossopharyngeal nerve

The glossopharyngeal nerve controls muscles of the pharynx and is sensory (including taste) to the caudal one third of the tongue and the pharyngeal mucosa [7,15]. It also innervates the parotid salivary gland by means of parasympathetic motor fibers [7]. The glossopharyngeal nerve arises from several roots extending from the lateral medulla in conjunction with the vagus and the accessory nerves [2,7]. CN IX exits the skull through the jugular foramen [3].

Vagus nerve

The vagus nerve is a mixed nerve providing motor innervation to the muscles of the pharynx and larynx and sensory innervation to the caudal pharynx, the larynx, and the abdominal viscera [7]. The vagus nerve also provides parasympathetic motor fibers to the thoracic and abdominal viscera. The vagus nerve arises from the lateral medulla in close association with CN IX and XI, and like other mammals, it exits the skull by means of the jugular foramen [3].

Accessory nerve

The accessory nerve is a pure motor nerve that innervates several muscles of the neck, including the cleidomastoid, sternomastoid, and trapezius muscles [2,7]. As with CN IX and CN X, the nerve roots arise from the lateral medulla; however, because this nerve is formed partially by cervical spinal nerves, the trunk of this nerve extends caudally on the spinal cord, so that its roots can arise as far back the fifth cervical spinal segment. There are approximately 10 accessory nerve roots in the rabbit [2,7]. The accessory nerve exits the skull by means of the jugular foramen [3].

Hypoglossal nerve

The hypoglossal nerve is a motor nerve that innervates the tongue and the hyoid muscles [2,7]. It arises from several roots located on the ventral surface of the caudal medulla at the lateral edge of the pyramids, similar in location to the ventral roots of a spinal nerve, and exits the skull by means of the hypoglossal canal [2,3].

Acknowledgments

The authors acknowledge the assistance of John Doval, Dr. William T. Ferrier, Susan Reiff, Dr. Jaromir Benak, Richard Larson, Jason Peters,

Winn Halina, Dr. Gary D. Partlow, Sam Tanng, Laura Cravens, and The Museum of Wildlife and Fish Biology UC Davis.

References

[1] Whitehouse R, Grove A. The dissection of the rabbit. London (UK): University Tutorial Press LTD; 1958.

[2] Craigie E. Practical anatomy of the rabbit. Toronto (Canada): University of Toronto Press; 1951.

[3] McLaughlin C, Chiasson R. Laboratory anatomy of the rabbit. 2nd edition. Dubuque (IA): William C Brown; 1979.

[4] Cruise L, Brewer N. Anatomy. The biology of the laboratory rabbit. San Diego (CA): Academic Press; 1994. p. 48–61.

[5] Greenaway J, Partlow G, Gonsholt N, et al. Anatomy of the lumbosacral spinal cord in rabbits. J Am Anim Hosp Assoc 2001;37:27–34.

[6] King AS. Physiological and clinical anatomy of the domestic mammals. vol. 1. Blackwell Science; 1987.

[7] Wingerd B, Stein G. Rabbit dissection manual. 1st edition. Baltimore (MD): The Johns Hopkins University Press; 1985.

[8] Kozma C, Macklin W, Cummins L, et al. Anatomy, physiology, and biochemistry of the rabbit. In: Weisbroth S, Flatt R, Kraus A, editors. The biology of the laboratory rabbit. New York: Academic Press; 1974. p. 50–72.

[9] Evans H. Miller's anatomy of the dog. 3rd edition. Philadelphia: W.B. Saunders Co.; 1993.

[10] Tencate J. Locomotory movements of the hind limbs in rabbits after isolation of the lumbosacral cord. J Exp Biol 1964;41:359–62.

[11] MacKay-Lyons M. Central pattern generation of locomotion: a review of the evidence. Phys Ther 2002;82(1):69–83.

[12] Laughton NB. Studies on the nervous regulation of progression in mammals. Am J Physiol 1924;70:358–84.

[13] Butler A. Comparative vertebrate neuroanatomy evolution and adaptation. 2nd edition. Hoboken (NJ): Wiley-Interscience; 2005.

[14] Hughes A. Topographical relationships between the anatomy and physiology of the rabbit visual system. Doc Ophthalmol 1971;30:33–159.

[15] Oliver J Jr, Lorenz M. Handbook of veterinary neurology. 2nd edition. Philadelphia: W.B. Saunders Co; 1993.

[16] Deeb B, Carpenter J. Neurologic and musculoskeletal diseases. In: Quesenberry K, Carpenter J, editors. Ferrets, rabbits, and rodents clinical medicine and surgery. 2nd edition. St. Louis (MO): Saunders; 2004. p. 203–10.

[17] Larsell O, Dow RS. The development of the cerebellum in the bat (Corynorhinus sp) and certain other mammals. J Comp Neurol 1935;1935(62):443–67.

[18] Voogd J, Wylie DR. Functional and anatomical organization of floccular zones: a preserved feature in vertebrates. J Comp Neurol 2004;470(2):107–12.

[19] Brown LT Jr. Projections and termination of the corticospinal tract in rodents. Exp Brain Res 1971;13(4):432–50.

[20] Murphy E, Garone M, Tashayyod D, et al. Innervation of the extraocular muscles of the rabbit. J Comp Neurol 1986;254:78–90.

[21] Popesko P, Rajtova V, Horak J. Colour atlas of the anatomy of small laboratory animals. Vol. 1: rabbit, guinea pig. St. Louis (MO): Saunders; 2002.

VETERINARY
CLINICS
Exotic Animal Practice

ELSEVIER
SAUNDERS

Vet Clin Exot Anim 10 (2007) 731–758

The Neurological Examination and Lesion Localization in the Companion Rabbit (*Oryctolagus cuniculus*)

Karen M. Vernau, DVM, MAS,
DACVIM (Neurology)[a],*,
Anna Osofsky, DVM, DABVP-Avian Practice[b],
Richard A. LeCouteur, BVSc, PhD,
DACVIM (Neurology)[a]

[a]*Department of Surgical and Radiological Sciences, School of Veterinary Medicine, University of California–Davis, Davis, CA, 95616, USA*
[b]*Carrollton West Pet Hospital, 3729 Old Denton Road, Carrollton, TX 75007, USA*

Completion of a thorough neurological examination is essential for clinicians to determine the location of a neurological problem in a rabbit. Together with history and signalment, determination of the location of a lesion (whether solitary or multifocal/diffuse) enables a clinician to list the most likely causes of the problem. Based on this list of differential diagnoses, a logical diagnostic plan is formed, leading to a diagnosis. Localization of a lesion(s) also allows targeting of appropriate diagnostic techniques (eg, computed tomography (CT) may be more appropriate when imaging bony structures of the middle ear in peripheral vestibular disease, versus magnetic resonance imaging (MRI) of the brainstem for animals with central vestibular disease). The significance of abnormalities defined by diagnostic tests is determined in part by the correlation with the clinical localization. In this article, the neurological examination of the rabbit is presented, followed by a practical guide to lesion localization in this species.

* Corresponding author.
E-mail address: kmvernau@ucdavis.edu (K.M. Vernau).

1094-9194/07/$ - see front matter © 2007 Elsevier Inc. All rights reserved.
doi:10.1016/j.cvex.2007.05.003 *vetexotic.theclinics.com*

Neurological examination

The neurological examination consists of a series of systematic observations of sensory and motor functions following naturally occurring or induced stimulation of the rabbit. The neurological examination is an extension of the general physical examination, and it should be completed only after the signalment (age, breed, sex, use of the animal), a complete and detailed history have been obtained, and a general physical examination have been completed.

General principles

Clinical neurology is based on a sound understanding of neuroanatomy, neurophysiology, and recognition of clinical signs resulting from loss of function of specific areas of the nervous system. A systematic and logical approach to the neurological examination permits a clinician to localize diseases to specific parts of the nervous system.

The objectives of the neurological examination are to detect the presence of a neurological abnormality and determine its location. This is called the neuroanatomical diagnosis. The neurological examination reflects only the location of the lesion. The signs seen at a given location will be the same regardless of the type of lesion. For example, trauma or an abscess may cause the same clinical signs if they occur in the same location.

A veterinarian must establish a routine standard procedure for examining a rabbit. This will provide the experience and confidence necessary to make an accurate neuroanatomical diagnosis. Results of the neurological examination should be carefully recorded progressively during the examination, and not left to memory. A neurological examination sheet should be used for this purpose (Fig. 1) and should be used for subsequent neurological examinations to allow the clinician to document the improvement or progression of disease. Only after the neurological examination has been completed, and the location(s) of a neurological abnormality determined, are ancillary diagnostic procedures (such as cerebrospinal fluid [CSF] examination or radiography) done to establish a diagnosis and decide on a treatment.

Approach to the neurological examination

The first step in locating a lesion is determining the level of the abnormality along the longitudinal plane of the neuroaxis.

The second step is to localize the lesion further within each of the following anatomical regions as follows:

- Brain—cerebral cortex, cerebellum, basal ganglia, brain stem, visual system, vestibular system
- Spinal cord—cranial cervical (Cl-C4), cervical enlargement (C5-T1), thoracolumbar (T2-L3), lumbosacral (L4-Cd+) [1]

- Peripheral nerve—peripheral nerve, dorsal root, ventral root, neuromuscular junction

The third step is to determine the location of the lesion in the transverse plane at the appropriate longitudinal level (eg, left or right side of the cerebral cortex).

RABBIT NEUROLOGICAL EXAMINATION FORM

Patient information   Examiner:_____

                                                          Date:_____

General Observations :

Mental status	bright/alert	obtunded	stuporous	comatose

Gait and Posture:

	Gait:	mono- -paresis ataxia	para- -plegia	tetra- circling	hemi-
	Posture:	Head		Trunk	Limbs

Cranial Nerves				**Postural Reactions**		
				CP:	LT	RT
					LP	LP
II:	Menace	OS	OD			
	Fundic	OS	OD	Wheelbarrow		
				Hopping	LT	RT
III:	Pupillary size	OS	OD		LP	RP
	PLR(direct)	OS	OD	Hemiwalking	L	R
	Consensual	OS	OD			
				Placing	Optic	
III,IV,VI:		OS	OD			
(tests: Observe for strabismus, physiological nystagmus, corneal reflex, pupil size)				Tactile		
				Righting reactions:		
V:	Motor	L	R	**Spinal Reflexes**		
	Sensory	Ophthal:	Ophthal:			
		Max:	Max:	Biceps	L:	R:
		Mand:	Mand:	Gastrocnemius	L:	R:
(tests: palpebral reflex, corneal reflex, jaw tone, lip pinch, masticatory muscle atrophy)						
VI:		L	R	Patellar	L:	R:
(tests: Observe for strabismus, physiological nystagmus, corneal re flex)						
VII		L	R			
(tests: facial symmetry, palpebral reflex)						
VIII:	Auditory	L	R	Triceps	L:	R:
	Head Tilt	L	R	Perineal		
	Nystagmus					
	Horizontal	Rotary	Vertical	Withdrawal	LT	RT
	Positional	Non-positional			RT	RP
	Fast-phase	L	R			

Fig. 1. Neurological examination form for the rabbit. *Abbreviations:* CP, conscious proprioception; L, left; PL, pelvic limb; R, right; TL, thoracic limb.

IX,X,XI: Crossed Extensor:
(tests: swallowing)

XII: Panniculus
(test: tongue movement, tongue atrophy)

Palpation
Musclemass/atrophy

Head palpation

Spinal palpation

Musculoskeletal examination

Assessment

1. Neurologically

      Normal   Abnormal

2. Neuroanatomical localization :

      Brain

      Spinal Cord

      Neuromuscular

3. Differential Diagnosis List

4. Diagnostic Plan

Fig. 1 (*continued*)

Conditions of the examination

Because rabbits are animals of prey, they are very nervous and may freeze during a neurological examination unless they are accustomed to being handled in this manner [2]. Rabbits must be handled carefully, not only to minimize their stress during the examination, but also to protect them from injury, such as spinal fractures, which may be caused by inappropriate or excessive restraint.

The neurological examination must be completed in a location free of distractions. Sedatives, narcotics, or tranquilizers should not be administered before the examination. It is important that the rabbit be as relaxed as possible.

Technique of the neurological examination

The neurological examination may be completed in any order. The following order of examination is recommended, as it starts with those parts of the examination that may be least likely to cause pain, and ends with those tests that may be either painful or may require close handling.

It is recommended that the neurological examination of the rabbit be completed in the following sequence:

- General observations
- Palpation
- Postural reactions
- Spinal reflexes
- Cranial nerves
- Sensation

General observations
Mental status. Allow the rabbit to move around the examination room while the examiner takes the history. Observe the rabbit's response to the environment.

Consciousness is a function of the cerebrum and brain stem (reticular formation). Sensory inputs from outside the body, for example light and sound, provide input to the reticular formation. Consciousness is maintained by diffuse projections of the reticular formation to the cerebral cortex. A common cause of decreased level of consciousness is disruption of these connections between the reticular formation and the cerebrum.

Mental status may be assessed as:

- Bright and alert (normal)
- Obtunded: conscious but inactive, unresponsive to the environment, tends to sleep when undisturbed
- Stuporous: sleeps when undisturbed, will not arouse to innocuous stimuli such as noise but will awaken with an apparently painful stimulus.
- Comatose: unconscious. The rabbit cannot be aroused even with a painful stimulus. Some simple reflexes may be intact. For example, pinching the foot may produce flexion of the limb but not arousal. Coma indicates complete disconnection of reticular formation and cerebrum.

Posture. Observe the rabbit while it is free to move about, and place the animal into different positions so that the ability to regain normal posture may be assessed.

Look for tilting of the head. Continuous tilting of the head usually is associated with an abnormality of vestibular function.

Abnormal posture of the trunk may be associated with congenital or acquired spinal cord lesions.

Abnormal postures and vertebral column include improper positioning of limbs, or increased or decreased extensor tone. Improper positioning of limbs (proprioceptive deficits) may result from a lesion anywhere in the neuraxis. Decreased tone of a limb usually results from a peripheral nerve lesion. Increased tone is a sign of spinal cord or brain disease (eg, decerebellate posture, decerebrate rigidity, or Schiff-Sherrington posture).

Gait. A nonslip surface is required for traction. Observe the rabbit from the side and moving toward and away from the examiner.

Neurological organization of gait and posture is complicated, involving brain, spinal cord and peripheral nerves. Normal rabbits use various gaits when moving slowly; however, most rabbits hop at faster speeds.

The assessment is determined as follows:

- Proprioception (position sense) is the ability to recognize the location of the limbs in relation to the rest of the body. A deficit is seen as knuckling or misplacement of the foot. Loss of proprioceptive positioning may be caused by a lesion at any level of the neuraxis, from the peripheral nerve to the cerebral cortex.
- Paresis is reduced voluntary movement. Plegia is absent voluntary movement. There may be monoparesis/plegia (one limb), paraparesis/paraplegia (both pelvic limbs), tetraparesis/plegia (all four limbs) or hemiparesis/plegia (thoracic and pelvic limbs on same side). Changes in voluntary movement are caused by disruption of the voluntary motor pathways that extend from the cerebral cortex, through the brain stem and spinal cord, to peripheral nerves.
- Ataxia is lack of coordination without paresis, spasticity, or involuntary movements (although each of these may be seen in association with ataxia). The movements of the limbs are uncoordinated, and feet may be crossed or placed too far apart. Ataxia may be caused by lesions at all levels of the neuraxis, but usually involves lesions of the cerebellum, vestibular system, or spinal cord.
- Dysmetria is characterized by movements that are too long (hypermetria) or short (hypometria). Hypermetria is more common, and most frequently is caused by a cerebellar lesion.
- Circling. Tight circles usually are caused by caudal brain stem lesions. The direction most often is toward the side of the lesion. A head tilt in association with circling usually indicates involvement of the vestibular system. Wide circles may be indicative of a lesion in the cerebrum or thalamus.

Palpation

The technique involves careful inspection and palpation of the bones, joints and muscles of the limbs, vertebral column and head. One side should be compared to the other to check for symmetry.

Assessment. Look for worn nails, masses, deviation of normal contour, abnormal motion, pain, or crepitation.

Evaluate size, tone, and strength of muscles. Muscle atrophy and loss of muscle strength usually accompany peripheral nerve diseases. Increased tone of extensor muscles is a common finding in brain and spinal cord diseases. Evaluation of muscle tone is done by passive stretch of a relaxed muscle. Rabbits rarely relax when being handled, thus accurate determination of muscle tone is extremely difficult. Determination of tail tone by manipulating the tail also may be possible.

Postural reactions

Postural reactions are the complex responses that maintain a rabbit's normal upright position and bring the limbs into an appropriate position to bear weight. These reactions consist of two phases. The first phase moves the foot into position and depends on the sensorimotor cortex (cerebral cortex) for recognition of the inappropriate foot position and initiation of the correcting movement. The second phase is the weight-bearing phase and depends on antigravity mechanisms in the brainstem and spinal cord. These reactions involve all levels of the nervous system; therefore, abnormalities of these reactions do not provide precise localizing information, as lesions of many different areas of the nervous system may affect these reactions.

Conscious proprioceptive positioning reactions. Flex the paw (each of the four limbs should be examined separately) so that the dorsal surface contacts the nonslip surface of the floor while supporting the rabbit underneath the thorax (to avoid bringing vestibular mechanisms into play). The rabbit should return the paw to a normal position immediately. In the authors' experience, most rabbits do not return the paw to the normal position unless they are very calm and are comfortable with being handled in this manner. Therefore, exercise caution in the interpretation of apparent conscious proprioceptive deficits in rabbits (Fig. 2).

Proprioceptive information is transmitted to the brain by means of the dorsal parts of the spinal cord. The motor response is initiated by the cerebrum, and is transmitted to the peripheral nerves by means of the spinal cord.

Delayed or absent correction may indicate an abnormality at any level of the nervous system, or may be normal in a nervous rabbit.

Wheelbarrowing reactions. The rabbit is supported under the abdomen with all weight on the thoracic limbs. The rabbit's lumbar vertebral column must be supported carefully during this test to avoid injury due to hyperextension. A normal rabbit will walk forward with coordinated movements of both thoracic limbs. This part of the examination should be attempted only with extremely calm rabbits to avoid injury. Provision of a mat or a surface that provides some traction will facilitate this test.

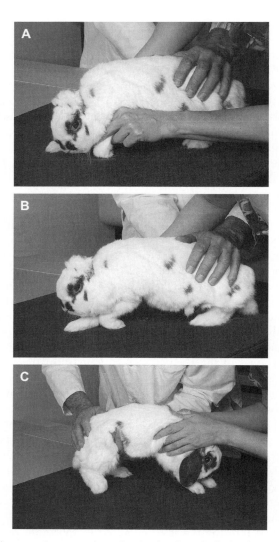

Fig. 2. (*A*) Testing conscious proprioception in the thoracic limb of a rabbit (*Oryctolagus cuniculus*). The left ear of this lop-eared rabbit has been moved gently to the right side to facilitate visualization. The rabbit is being examined on a nonslip surface by the examiner and an assistant. The examiner is supporting the rabbit under the thorax, while the left thoracic limb is turned so that the dorsal surface of the paw is resting on the mat. The assistant is supporting the dorsal lumbar area of the rabbit. (*B*) Testing conscious proprioception in the thoracic limb of a rabbit (*Oryctolagus cuniculus*). The examiner's hand has been removed from the left thoracic limb, but continues to support the rabbit under the thorax. Note that the left thoracic limb remains knuckled in this neurologically normal rabbit. Although this is not a normal finding, because rabbits are prey animals, some rabbits may freeze during the examination and display conscious proprioceptive deficits. (*C*) Testing conscious proprioception in the pelvic limb of a rabbit (*Oryctolagus cuniculus*). Note that the rabbit is being examined on a nonslip mat by an examiner and assistant. The examiner is supporting the rabbit under the abdomen and supports the lumbar vertebral column, while the paw is turned on the dorsal surface. Note the apparent deficit of conscious proprioception in this neurologically normal rabbit.

Slow initiation of movement may be a sign of a lesion in the cervical spinal cord, brain stem, or cerebral cortex. Exaggerated movements (dysmetria) may indicate an abnormality in the cervical spinal cord, lower brain stem, or cerebellum.

Hopping reactions. The hopping reactions of the thoracic limbs are tested with the rabbit in position for wheelbarrowing but with one thoracic limb lifted from the ground. The entire weight is supported on one limb, and the rabbit is moved laterally. The hopping reaction of the pelvic limbs is completed similarly (Fig. 3).

Hopping reactions are more sensitive than the wheelbarrowing reaction for detecting minor deficits. Abnormalities may be caused by lesions at all levels of the neuraxis. Poor initiation of the hopping reaction suggests

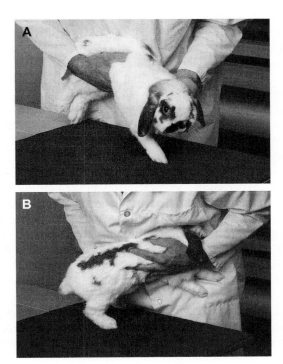

Fig. 3. (*A*) Evaluation of hopping reaction in the thoracic limb of a rabbit (*Oryctolagus cuniculus*). The rabbit is examined on a nonslip surface. The rabbit's thorax is being supported ventrally by the examiner with the same hand that is keeping the left thoracic limb in flexion. The pelvic limbs are lifted off the ground with the examiner's other hand, which restrains the pelvic limbs and pelvis against the examiner's body. The rabbit is hopped laterally, away from the examiner. (*B*) Evaluation of hopping reaction in the pelvic limb of a rabbit (*Oryctolagus cuniculus*). The rabbit is examined on a nonslip surface. The rabbit's abdomen is being supported ventrally by the examiner with the same hand that is keeping the right pelvic limb in flexion. The thoracic limbs are lifted off the ground with the examiner's other hand, which restrains thorax and head against the examiner's body. The rabbit is hopped laterally, away from the examiner.

sensory (proprioceptive) deficits, whereas poor movement suggests a motor system abnormality. Asymmetry may help to lateralize a lesion.

Hemistanding and hemiwalking reactions. Thoracic and pelvic limbs of one side are lifted from the ground so that all of the rabbit's weight is supported by the opposite limbs. Then lateral walking movements are evaluated.

Assessment is the same as for other postural reactions.

Placing reactions. Placing is evaluated first without vision (tactile placing) and then with vision (visual placing). The examiner supports the rabbit under the thorax and covers the eyes with one hand or with a blindfold. The thoracic limbs are brought in contact with the edge of a table at or below the carpus. The normal response is immediate placement of the paws on the table surface in a position that will support weight. Care must be taken not to restrict the movement of either limb. When one limb is consistently slower to respond, the animal should be held on the other side of the examiner to ensure that movements are not being restricted. Visual and tactile placing reactions are difficult to elicit in the pelvic limbs. Visual placing is tested by allowing the rabbit to see the table surface. Normal animals reach for the surface before the carpus touches the table. Placing reactions may be difficult to elicit in rabbits that are nervous; therefore, care must be taken in their interpretation.

Tactile placing requires integrity of touch receptors in the skin, sensory pathways through the spinal cord and the brain stem to the cerebral cortex, and motor pathways from the cerebral cortex to the peripheral nerves of the thoracic limbs. Visual placing requires integrity of visual pathways to the cerebral cortex, communication from the visual cortex to the motor cortex, and motor pathways to the peripheral nerves of the thoracic limbs.

A lesion of any portion of the pathways may cause a deficit in placing reactions. Normal tactile placing with absent visual placing indicates a lesion in the visual system. Normal visual placing with abnormal tactile placing suggests a sensory pathway lesion. Cortical lesions may produce a deficit in the contralateral limbs, whereas lesions caudal to the midbrain usually produce ipsilateral motor deficits in the limbs. Neurologically normal rabbits may have placing reaction deficits secondary to their response to stress.

Righting reactions. Place and hold the rabbit on its side, then release and observe its ability to rise. Make sure that the lumbar vertebral column is supported appropriately to prevent hyperextension. Once again, this part of the examination should be performed only in tractable rabbits, as lateral recumbency is not a normal posture for an animal that is predated upon by carnivorous species. Note that righting of the head and not the body may indicate cervical spinal cord disease.

Tonic neck reactions. These reactions are difficult to elicit and interpret in rabbits, and they usually are not examined.

Spinal reflexes

Examination of spinal reflexes tests the integrity of the sensory and motor components of the reflex arc and the influence of descending motor pathways on the reflexes.

Phasic stretch reflexes. Percussion of a muscle belly (eg, extensor carpi radialis or cranial tibial muscles) may elicit a phasic stretch reflex, but also may cause muscle contraction by direct stimulation of excitable muscle fibers. Therefore, this method of eliciting tendon reflexes is not as useful or reliable as actually striking a tendon directly.

There are three categories of reflexes:

1. Absence or depression of a reflex indicates complete or partial loss of either the sensory or motor nerves responsible for the reflex.
2. A normal reflex indicates that the sensory and motor nerves are intact.
3. An exaggerated reflex indicates an abnormality in the descending pathways from the brain that normally have a predominantly inhibitory influence on reflex arcs.

Spinal reflex examinations should be performed with the rabbit in lateral recumbency if the rabbit will tolerate being held in this position without undue stress.

The uppermost limbs should be examined, and the rabbit should be rolled to the opposite side to complete examination of the contralateral limbs. Muscle tone (previously evaluated with the rabbit in a standing position) should be assessed again at this time. Pelvic limbs reflexes usually are evaluated before thoracic limb reflexes.

Patellar (knee-jerk, quadriceps) reflex. With the rabbit in lateral recumbency, the uppermost pelvic limb is supported under the femur with the left hand and the stifle is flexed slightly. The straight patellar ligament is struck crisply with a reflex hammer. The reflex is seen as a single, rapid extension of the stifle (Fig. 4).

The myotatic reflexes are basic to the regulation of posture and movement. The reflex arc is a simple, two-neuron (monosynaptic) pathway.

The patellar reflex is the most reliably interpreted myotatic reflex. The reflex should be recorded as absent (0), depressed (1+), normal (2+), exaggerated (3+), or exaggerated with clonus (4+).

Absence of a myotatic reflex indicates a lesion of the sensory or motor (lower motor neuron) component of the reflex arc. Loss of the reflex in one muscle group suggests a peripheral nerve lesion (ie, of the femoral nerve). Bilateral loss of the reflex suggests a segmental spinal cord lesion affecting the motor neurons to both pelvic limbs located in spinal cord

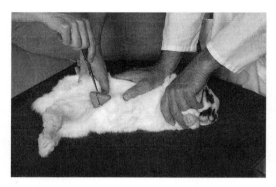

Fig. 4. Evaluation of the patellar reflex during a neurological examination of a rabbit (*Orycto-lagus cuniculus*). The rabbit is examined by the examiner and an assistant. The assistant restrains the thoracic limbs and head with one hand, while gently supporting the lumbar vertebral column with the other hand. The examiner strikes the patellar tendon of the uppermost limb and assesses the degree of extension of the limb.

segments L4 to L6 (in rabbits with 12 thoracic and seven lumbar vertebrae) and L3 to L5 (in rabbits with 13 thoracic and six lumbar vertebrae) [3]. Depression of the reflex has the same significance as absence of the reflex except that the causative lesion is incomplete. Exaggerated reflexes and increased tone result from loss of descending inhibitory pathways from the brain in the spinal cord cranial to the L4 to L6 (or L3 to L5) spinal cord segments.

Triceps reflex. The rabbit is placed into lateral recumbency, and the thoracic limb is supported under the elbow with flexion of the elbow and the carpus maintained. The tendon of insertion of the triceps brachii muscle is struck with a reflex hammer just proximal to the olecranon. The reflex is seen as a slight extension of the elbow. Contraction of the triceps muscle also may be noted.

The triceps brachii muscle extends the elbow, and it is essential for weight bearing in the thoracic limb. Innervation is by the radial nerve with its origin in spinal cord segments C7–T1 (canine spinal cord segments listed as data concerning the anatomy of the brachial enlargement and muscular innervation are lacking in rabbits).

The triceps reflex is difficult to elicit in the normal rabbit. Absent or decreased reflexes should not always be interpreted as abnormal. Exaggerated reflexes are indicative of a lesion cranial to C7.

Biceps reflex. The index or middle finger of the examiner's hand that is holding the rabbit's elbow is placed on the biceps and the brachialis tendons cranial and proximal to the elbow. The elbow is extended slightly, and the finger is struck with the reflex hammer. The reflex is seen as a slight flexion of the elbow and contraction of the biceps muscle.

The biceps brachii muscle is a flexor of the elbow and is innervated by the musculocutaneous nerve that originates from spinal cord segments C6 to C8 (in the dog).

The biceps reflex is difficult to elicit in the normal rabbit. An exaggerated reflex is indicative of a lesion cranial to C6.

Flexion reflexes. The rabbit is maintained in lateral recumbency, with the lumbar vertebral column supported to prevent hyperextension. A sensory stimulus is applied to the foot. The normal reflex is flexion of the entire limb, followed by an immediate relaxation of the limb. The least sensory stimulus necessary to elicit flexion should be used. The stimulus should be removed immediately after flexion begins (Fig. 5).

The flexion reflex involves all the flexor muscles of the limb being tested and thus requires activation of motor neurons in several spinal cord segments. The flexion reflex is a spinal reflex and does not require any activation of the brain.

The pelvic limb flexion reflex primarily involves spinal cord segments L6–S2 and the sciatic nerve [3]. Absence or depression of the reflex indicates a lesion of these spinal cord segments or nerves. Unilateral absence of the reflex is more likely the result of a peripheral nerve lesion, whereas bilateral absence or depression of the reflex is more likely the result of a spinal cord or cauda equina lesion. A normal flexion reflex indicates that the segments and the nerves are functional. An exaggerated flexion reflex usually reflects a (chronic) lesion cranial to L6.

Flexor muscles of the thoracic limbs are innervated by the axillary, musculocutaneous, median and ulnar nerves, and by parts of the radial nerve. Discrepancy exists in what is reported for the spinal cord segments

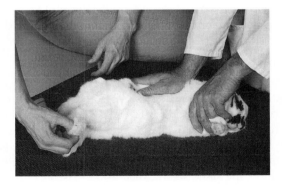

Fig. 5. Assessment of the withdrawal reflex in the pelvic limb of a rabbit (*Oryctolagus cuniculus*). The rabbit is examined by the examiner and an assistant. The assistant restrains the thoracic limbs and head with one hand, while gently supporting the lumbar vertebral column with the other hand. The examiner starts with a gentle but noxious stimulus to the skin of the pelvic limb toes in the up limb and assesses the degree of flexion of the limb.

that form the brachial intumescence and the spinal nerve contributions to the peripheral nerves of the thoracic limb. Different authors report spinal nerve contributions to be C4–T1 [2,4] or C5–T1 [1] in the rabbit. The authors believe that there is a paucity of anatomical research in this area, and thus the information that is published in textbooks is not scientifically validated. Therefore, the authors do not know what constitutes the brachial intumescence or plexus in the rabbit. Thus for this article, the brachial plexus will be referred to as C6–T2 based on information from dogs [5].

The axillary, musculocutaneous, median, and ulnar nerves originate from spinal cord segments C6–T1, with small contributions from C5 and T2. Depressed reflexes indicate a lesion of these spinal cord segments, or of the peripheral nerves. Exaggeration of thoracic limb reflexes indicates a lesion cranial to C6.

Perineal (anal) reflex. The perineal reflex is elicited by light stimulation of the perineum with a needle, cotton-tipped applicator, or forceps. The reflex is seen as a contraction of the anal sphincter muscle.

Sensory innervation occurs through the pudendal nerve and spinal cord segments S2 and S3 [3]. Motor innervation of the anal sphincter also occurs through the pudendal nerve. The organization of the reflex is similar to that of the flexion reflex.

The perineal reflex provides an indication of the functional integrity of the sacral spinal cord segments and the sacral nerve roots. Evaluation of this reflex is especially important in rabbits with urinary bladder dysfunction. Absence or depression of the reflex indicates a sacral spinal cord lesion or a pudendal nerve lesion.

Crossed extensor reflex. The crossed extensor reflex may be observed when the flexor reflex is elicited. The response is an extension of the limb opposite to the stimulated limb. This reflex is not observed in normal animals in a clinical setting. This reflex may be observed best by eliciting a withdrawal reflex of the lowermost limb and observing for extension of the uppermost limb.

Crossed extensor reflexes result from lesions affecting descending inhibitory pathways of the spinal cord. The crossed extensor reflex is considered evidence of a severe spinal cord lesion.

Note that the spinal thrust reflex (rapid caudal movement of a pelvic limb) or mass reflex (simultaneous movement of tail, anal sphincter, both pelvic limbs) may be seen in the pelvic limbs when attempting a flexor reflex. These reflexes have the same significance as a crossed extensor reflex.

Cranial nerves

Examination of cranial nerves is an important part of the neurological examination, especially when a brain lesion is suspected.

Olfaction. The olfactory nerve (cranial nerve I) is the sensory pathway for the conscious perception of smell.

A behavioral response to a pleasurable or noxious odor may be used.

Chemoreceptors in the nasal mucosa give rise to axons that pass through the cribriform plate to synapse in the olfactory bulb. Axons from the olfactory bulb course through the olfactory tract, mostly to the ipsilateral olfactory cortex.

Deficiencies in the sense of smell are difficult to evaluate, and this test is not done routinely in rabbits.

Vision. The optic nerve (cranial nerve II) is the sensory pathway for vision and pupillary light reflexes.

The optic nerve is tested by means of three major tests:

1. Menace response. The examiner elicits the menace reaction by making a threatening gesture with the hand at one eye, being careful to avoid touching the sensory hairs of the eyelids, and avoiding creation of wind currents. The normal response is a blink and sometimes an aversive movement of the head. Because rabbits are nervous animals that often freeze during the examination, many rabbits do not respond to the menace response (that is, they do not blink when a threatening gesture is made toward the eye).
2. Visual placing reaction.
3. Ophthalmoscopic examination. Abnormalities of the eye may affect vision, the menace response, and the pupillary light reflexes.

Lesions from the retina to the cerebral cortex (contralateral) may result in a menace reaction deficit. Because many neurologically normal rabbits may have an absent menace response, care must be taken when interpreting a negative response.

Pupil size and response (cranial nerves II and III). The oculomotor nerve (cranial nerve III) contains the parasympathetic motor fibers for pupillary constriction. It also is the motor pathway for several extraocular eye muscles and for the levator muscle of the upper eyelid.

The examiner shines a light into each eye, and observes pupillary constriction in both eyes.

Observe the pupils for size and symmetry. Both pupils should constrict when a light is shined into either eye.

Bilateral, widely dilated pupils may result from excessive sympathetic influences (eg, fear, excitement), or from lack of parasympathetic innervation (cranial nerve III). A unilateral lesion of the midbrain or oculomotor nerve may cause a dilated and unresponsive pupil on the same side as the lesion (this may be differentiated from optic nerve diseases because the eye will have vision).

Bilaterally constricted pupils may result from excessive parasympathetic influence (eg, organophosphate poisoning). A unilaterally constricted pupil may be due to a lesion of the sympathetic innervation to the pupil (Horner's syndrome).

Extraocular positioning and movements (cranial nerves III–VI). Observe the eyes with the head not moving and with the head in various positions to check for symmetrical positioning of the eyes, strabismus (abnormal deviation), and resting nystagmus. The latter two are abnormal. Move the head from side to side and up and down and observe for vestibular nystagmus, the normal (physiological) nystagmus seen with head movement.

Oculomotor nerve (cranial nerve III) is the motor pathway for the dorsal, medial and ventral rectus, and ventral oblique muscles. Trochlear nerve (cranial nerve IV) is the motor pathway for the dorsal oblique muscle. The abducens nerve (cranial nerve VI) innervates the lateral rectus and retractor bulbi muscles. For vestibular nystagmus to be present, the vestibular system, the brain stem (medial longitudinal fasciculus) and cranial nerves III, IV, and VI must be functioning normally.

The eyes should move in coordination with each other (conjugate eye movements).

Lesions of the oculomotor nerve cause a fixed lateral deviation (strabismus) of the eye, inability to move the eye medially, ptosis, and a dilated pupil on the side ipsilateral to the lesion.

Lesions of the trochlear nerve cause a lateral rotation of the eye that is most apparent in cats (which have a vertical pupil). Lesions of the abducens nerve cause a loss of lateral gaze, medial strabismus, and an inability to retract the globe.

Trigeminal nerve (cranial nerve V). The trigeminal nerve is the motor pathway to the muscles of mastication and the sensory pathway to the face (eyelids, cornea, oral cavity, and mucosa of internal nares).

Motor function is tested by assessing for atrophy of the muscles of mastication and jaw tone. It is more difficult to examine jaw tone in rabbits than in other domestic species. Compared with carnivorous animal species, rabbits have a very small mouth opening, and their oral cavity is long and narrow. Thus, gaining access to the oral cavity and assessing jaw tone are more challenging in rabbits. A small syringe case or small tongue depressor may be placed into the mouth behind the incisors to evaluate jaw tone. Sensory function is tested by checking for sensation over the face (Fig. 6), nasal mucosa (Fig. 7), and cornea (Fig. 8).

The motor branch of cranial nerve V is in the mandibular nerve, which innervates the masseter, temporal, rostral digastricus, pterygoid, and myelohyoid muscles (canine data is listed here as information concerning the anatomy is lacking in rabbits). All three branches of the trigeminal nerve

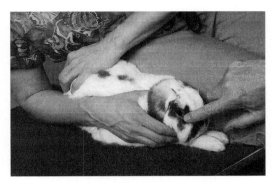

Fig. 6. Evaluation of the palpebral reflex during a neurological examination of a rabbit (*Oryctolagus cuniculus*). The rabbit is examined by the examiner and an assistant. The examiner touches the medial and lateral canthus of each eye and assesses the resultant blink.

(ophthalmic, maxillary, and mandibular) are sensory. These branches collectively innervate the face, lips, nasal mucosa, and cornea. Sensory function may be evaluated by monitoring facial nerve function (ie, blink reflex: sensory is cranial nerve V; motor is cranial nerve VII) and abducens nerve function (ie, corneal reflex: sensory is cranial nerve V; motor is cranial nerve VI) in response to sensory stimulation of the face and the cornea, respectively.

Bilateral disorders of the mandibular branch of cranial nerve V may cause a dropped jaw, which may be difficult to appreciate in a rabbit. Unilateral lesions result in decreased jaw tone. Atrophy of the temporal and masseter muscles may be recognized.

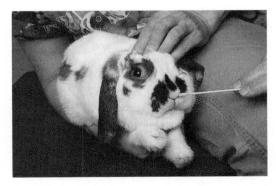

Fig. 7. Evaluation of nasal sensation during a neurological examination of a rabbit (*Oryctolagus cuniculus*). The rabbit is examined by the examiner and an assistant. The soft end of a cotton-tipped applicator is used to stimulate the nasal mucosa of the left and right side of the nasal cavity. A normal response is to withdraw the head. Rabbits that are very nervous may not respond to this test of nasal sensation.

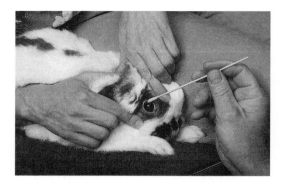

Fig. 8. Evaluation of the corneal reflex during a neurological examination of a rabbit (*Oryctolagus cuniculus*). The examiner uses a moist cotton-tipped applicator to gently touch the cornea, while the assistant restrains the rabbit. When the cornea is touched, the eye is retracted into the orbit, and the rabbit may (or may not) blink.

Facial nerve (cranial nerve VII). The facial nerve is motor to the muscles of facial expression and the sensory pathway for taste to the palate and rostral two-thirds of the tongue. Additionally, it supplies all major exocrine glands of the head (lacrimation and salivation), except parotid and zygomatic salivary glands.

Note facial symmetry (Fig. 9). Check for ability to move ears and blink (V–VII reflexes). Because rabbits produce a low volume of tears, lacrimal secretions are evaluated best with the phenol red thread test rather than the Schirmir Tear Test [6].

Asymmetry of the face usually is seen in facial paralysis (lips, eyelids, and ears may droop), with blink reflexes absent and no response to taste testing (Fig. 10).

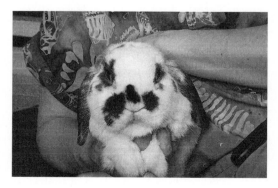

Fig. 9. Evaluating facial symmetry of a rabbit (*Oryctolagus cuniculus*). The examiner should evaluate the character and symmetry of ear carriage, eye position in the orbit, eyelids, nose, and lips.

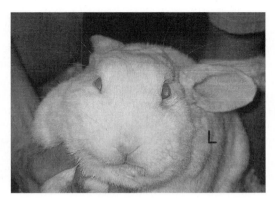

Fig. 10. A rabbit (*Oryctolagus cuniculus*) with left facial paralysis. Note the drooping left ear, wider left palpebral fissure, droopy left lip, and saliva staining around the mouth.

Vestibulocochlear nerve (cranial nerve VIII). The vestibulocochlear nerve has two divisions. The cochlear division mediates hearing, and the vestibular division provides information about the orientation of the head with respect to gravity (equilibrium, balance).

Both hearing and vestibular function should be evaluated:

- Hearing. Evaluate the rabbit's behavioral response to sound. Partial or unilateral hearing loss may be difficult to evaluate clinically.
- Vestibular function: (partially evaluated in the examination of gait and posture). Observe for head tilt, strabismus, ataxia, or nystagmus (Fig. 11).

Unilateral vestibulocochlear nerve disease may produce head tilt, circling, positional strabismus, spontaneous nystagmus, and loss of hearing.

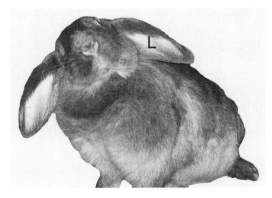

Fig. 11. A rabbit (*Oryctolagus cuniculus*) with a right-sided head tilt caused by peripheral vestibular disease.

Glossopharyngeal nerve (cranial nerve IX) and vagus nerve (cranial nerve X) (swallowing). The swallowing reflex is elicited by gentle external pressure on the hyoid region and observing the rabbit swallowing. This reflex is difficult to elicit in nervous rabbits. The gag reflex cannot be done in rabbits because of the anatomy of their oral cavity.

Nuclei of both nerves are located in the caudal medulla. The glossopharyngeal nerve is the motor pathway to the muscles of the pharynx, and the vagus nerve is the motor pathway to the pharynx and the larynx. The vagus nerve is the sensory pathway to the caudal pharynx and larynx.

Hypoglossal nerve (cranial nerve XII). Wet the rabbit's nose and observe its ability to extend the tongue. The mouth also may be opened carefully with a small syringe case or tongue depressor, and the tongue may be observed for atrophy. Tongue strength is difficult to evaluate in rabbits, because their tongues are difficult to grasp. Care must be taken not to overextend the tongue or inadvertent laceration of the tongue on the mandibular incisors may occur.

Sensation

Observations of body sensation basically are limited to observations of proprioception (position sense) and nociception (pain perception). Evaluation of mechanoreception is problematic, because even normal animals may not respond to non-noxious mechanical stimulation of the skin. If the rabbit does not respond to a stimulus, then a stronger stimulus may be required, possibly even a noxious stimulus, to ascertain sensory function.

At this point in the neurological examination, sensation has been tested by assessment of the cranial nerves, the spinal reflexes, and proprioceptive positioning. Sensory modalities still to be tested include superficial pain perception and deep pain perception from limbs and trunk.

Technique. Begin caudally and progress cranially. Start with minimal stimulus and slowly increase strength until the rabbit shows evidence of cerebral perception (eg, turning toward stimulus, struggling). A significant behavioral response indicates the presence of sensation. Pain perception may be difficult to interpret in rabbits, because they may freeze and not respond, even to a painful stimulus. Repeating the examination or pain perception test may be useful in some rabbits. It also may be necessary to test pain perception in a limb that should not be involved in the neurological problem (eg, the thoracic limb skin when the lesion has been localized to a T3–L3 myelopathy. The thoracic limb should be normal. If the rabbit does not respond to pinching the thoracic limb, then the response in the pelvic limb cannot be interpreted).

Superficial pain perception is tested by squeezing the skin. If superficial pain sensation is present, testing for deep pain perception is not necessary.

Deep pain perception is tested by squeezing deeper structures (eg, bones and periosteum of the digits) using an instrument such as a hemostat.

Withdrawal of the limb alone does not confirm conscious pain perception. This is a segmental spinal reflex.

A conscious response (eg, turning of the head) implies intact conscious pain perception (ie, sensory information is able to ascend the spinal cord to the brain, past the area of damaged spinal cord).

The cutaneous trunci reflex (or panniculus reflex) is a twitching of the cutaneous trunci muscles of the back in response to cutaneous stimulation. This is a bilateral reflex, stronger on the side of the stimulus.

Assessment. Alterations in sensation are described as absent (0), decreased (1+), normal (2+), and increased (3+). Absent or decreased sensation indicates damage to a sensory nerve or a central pathway. Increased sensitivity may indicate irritation of a nerve.

Lesions of a peripheral nerve produce a pattern of abnormality conforming to the sensory distribution of that particular peripheral nerve.

Loss of function in the limbs caudal to a spinal cord lesion develops (and returns in the reverse order) in the following sequence:

1. Loss of proprioception
2. Altered voluntary motor function
3. Loss of superficial pain sensation
4. Loss of deep pain sensation

Therefore, an animal with a spinal cord compression that has lost proprioception and voluntary motor function (paralysis), but still has superficial and deep pain sensation, has less severe spinal cord damage than one that has lost all four functions. A loss of deep pain perception indicates a severely damaged spinal cord and consequently a poor prognosis.

Loss of deep pain perception is an extremely important clinical sign relating to prognosis. It implies severe and extensive damage to the spinal cord sufficient to damage even the most resilient nerve fibers. Prolonged absence of deep pain perception (>24 hours) carries a poor prognosis, as does loss of deep pain associated with traumatic injuries such as vertebral fractures/luxations.

It is imperative to be able to assess pain perception in an animal, and to be able to differentiate between an unconscious reflex withdrawal of a limb and conscious pain perception.

Localization of neurological disease

Once the rabbit's signalment and history are known, and physical and neurological examinations have been completed, a clinician must determine if there is a neurological problem. Once the rabbit is assessed as having a neurological problem, the next step is to localize the problem to a specific area within the nervous system. The following discussion will help a clinician to evaluate abnormal findings of the rabbit's neurological examination so that the lesion may be localized.

General localization of brain disease

Rabbits with brain disease may have altered mentation and/or behavior changes such as aggression. When they have cerebral or thalamic disease, they may complete wide, compulsive circles; tight circles may be seen with brainstem disease. Postural reactions are difficult to interpret in rabbits, because many normal rabbits will apparently exhibit postural reaction deficits. Rabbits with brainstem disease may have ipsilateral postural reaction deficits, whereas rabbits with thalamic or cerebral disease may have contralateral deficits. Rabbits with cerebral disease may have contralateral hemiparesis; with brainstem disease they may have ipsilateral hemiparesis. Animals with brainstem disease may have cranial nerve deficits such as facial paralysis and vestibular dysfunction. Rabbits with cerebral cortical disease may have seizures.

Upper and lower motor neurons

Upper motor neurons (UMNs) are neurons that originate in motor areas of the brain. They travel down the spinal cord and synapse, by means of interneurons, with the lower motor neurons (LMNs). UMNs are essential for the initiation of voluntary movement, and they also have an important role in moderating the tonic activity of the LMNs.

LMNs have the cell bodies in the ventral horn of the gray matter, the axons run in the ventral nerve root and peripheral nerve, and supplies the appropriate muscles. The LMN, its axon and the muscle fibers supplied comprise the motor unit. The LMN is the final common pathway for motor activity, whether this is under the direction of the higher centers in the brain by means of UMN (voluntary), or local reflex pathways. The assessment of reflexes (particularly limb reflexes) is an important component of the neurological examination, and it is especially helpful in determining the presence or absence of UMN or LMN lesions. The means to differentiate between UMN and LMN is listed in Table 1.

Motor function. Decreased (paresis) or absent (paralysis) voluntary movement can result from lesions affecting both UMNs (loss of signals initiating movement) and LMNs (loss of the effectors of movement). Therefore, paresis/paralysis does not help to differentiate a UMN lesion from a LMN lesion.

Muscle tone. Tonic activity of LMNs is responsible for resting muscle tone. Loss of the LMN will result in decreased/absent muscle tone. Many UMNs have an inhibitory influence on LMN and resting muscle tone. UMN lesions may result in increased muscle tone.

Table 1
Differentiating upper and lower motor neuron lesions

	Lower motor neuron lesion (partial–complete)	Upper motor neuron lesion (partial–complete)
Motor function	Paresis to paralysis	Paresis to paralysis
Local reflexes	Decreased to absent	Present (may be increased)
Muscle tone	Decreased to absent	Present (may be increased)
Muscle atrophy	Moderate to severe	Minimal

Local reflexes. Limb reflexes, such as tendon reflexes and flexion reflexes, as well as nonlimb reflexes such as the perineal reflex, are mediated at the segmental spinal cord level by means of LMNs. Loss of LMNs will result in decreased/absent reflexes. As with muscle tone, the UMN may modulate the nature of the reflex. UMN lesions do not result in loss of reflexes. Reflexes may be exaggerated with an UMN lesion.

Atrophy. Loss of LMNs will result in profound neurogenic atrophy (denervation) of the muscle fibers supplied by that nerve. Atrophy usually is apparent within 7 days. UMN lesions causing paresis/paralysis may result in minimal muscle atrophy secondary to disuse; however, if the LMNs are intact, profound atrophy will not be present.

Cutaneous trunci reflex. The panniculus or cutaneous trunci reflex is mediated by the lateral thoracic nerve, which originates from the brachial plexus and receives nerve fibers from C8–T1 spinal cord segments [7]. The afferent input is organized on a dermatomal basis with inputs bilaterally at segmental levels from about L7.

Lesions affecting C8–T1 cord segments (or nerve roots) will result in loss of the reflex regardless of the site of stimulation. T3–L3 spinal cord lesions will result in loss of the reflex caudal to the last intact dermatome. The level of cut-off therefore may be used to more accurately localize lesions within the T3–L3 region. The cutaneous trunci reflex may remain intact with mild-to-moderate spinal cord lesions, and it can be inconsistent in some rabbits.

Sympathetic function. Central sympathetic fibers descend in the lateral columns of the spinal cord and synapse with preganglionic neurons in the lateral gray matter of TI–L5. Cervical lesions may cause loss of vascular tone and skin hyperthermia affecting the head, body, and limbs. Horner's syndrome may be seen with cervical lesions, or more commonly T1–T3 lesions, particularly those affecting the lateral columns and lateral gray matter.

Schiff-Sherrington posture. Severe damage to the thoracic or lumbar spinal cord can result in marked increase in thoracic limb extensor tone with rigid extension of the thoracic limbs. This is caused by interruption of ascending inhibitory pathways from cells located in the lumbar spinal cord segments (so-called border cells). Schiff-Sherrington posture usually is an indicator of a poor prognosis, particularly if present for prolonged periods (>24 hours). Voluntary movement, reflexes, and proprioception are normal in the thoracic limbs, but may appear abnormal because of the increased muscle tone. Painful spinal cord lesions also may result in animals adopting a rigid thoracic limb posture unrelated to the Schiff-Sherrington posture. Animals with Schiff-Sherrington posture usually have paraplegia without deep pain perception in the pelvic limbs. When transient, it is not necessarily associated with a grave prognosis.

Abnormal respiration. Damage to descending respiratory pathways (reticulospinal tracts) from the medullary respiratory centers, to the motor neurons of the phrenic nerve (C4-7), or to intercostal nerves (T1 to T13) may result in respiratory insufficiency. Paradoxical respiration with inward movement of the chest wall may be seen if most intercostal muscles are paralyzed and diaphragmatic function (phrenic nerve) is maintained. Respiratory compromise is seen most commonly with severe high cervical lesions (probably because of involvement of descending UMNs), or with severe motor unit disease.

General localization of spinal cord disease

Spinal cord disease is localized to one of four anatomical regions of the spinal cord:

- C1 to C5—descending UMN to thoracic limb and pelvic limb; ascending sensory fibers from thoracic and pelvic limbs
- C6–T2 (Cervical enlargement)—descending UMN to pelvic limbs and LMN to thoracic limb; ascending sensory fibers from thoracic and pelvic limbs
- T3–L3—descending UMN to pelvic limb; ascending sensory fibers from pelvic limb
- L4–caudal (lumbar enlargement)—LMN to pelvic limb (bladder and tail); ascending sensory fibers from pelvic limb

Localization of a lesion in the spinal cord

Determine which limbs are affected (eg, are all four limbs involved, or just the pelvic limbs?). This is done by assessing gait, voluntary movement, and postural reactions If the thoracic limbs are normal, the lesion is caudal to the T2 spinal cord segment. If the thoracic limbs are abnormal, the lesion is cranial to T2 spinal cord segment.

Determine whether LMN signs are present in the affected limbs.

Use the presence/absence of LMN signs in the affected limbs to logically localize the lesion. UMN signs thoracic and pelvic limbs indicate C1-C5 myelopathy. LMN signs in the thoracic limbs and UMN signs in the pelvic limbs indicate a C6-T2 myelopathy. Normal thoracic limbs and UMN signs in the pelvic limbs indicate a T3–L3 myelopathy. Normal thoracic limbs and LMN signs in the pelvic limbs (and/or bladder, tail) indicate a L4–caudal myelopathy.

Two lesions between T3 and L3 may result in similar clinical signs as a solitary T3–L3 lesion.

LMN signs from a lesion in the lumbar enlargement (paraparesis, hyporeflexia, hypotonia) may mask the clinical signs of a second T3–L3 lesion (paraparesis, normal/exaggerated tone, reflexes).

With respect to UMN and LMN signs, brain disease usually results in UMN signs in all four limbs or in both thoracic and pelvic limbs on the same side.

General localization of neuromuscular disease

Rabbits with neuromuscular disease may have generalized weakness, gait abnormalities, and exercise-related weakness. They may have paresis/paralysis of the limbs and cranial nerves. They may have signs of dysphagia, dyspnea, profound muscle atrophy, or skeletal deformities. Rabbits with neuromuscular disease frequently may have LMN signs in all four limbs.

Diagnostic plan for rabbits with neurological disease

Clinicians should be aware of the most common neurological diseases recognized in rabbits, to effect timely diagnosis and treatment of rabbits in their care.

A minimum database (complete blood count [CBC]; serum biochemistry analysis, including creatine kinase; urinalysis; thoracic; and/or abdominal radiographic/ultrasound studies) should be considered in most rabbits with neurological disease to identify systemic disease, and/or concurrent disease. Rabbits with a history of trauma should be manipulated as minimally as possible to avoid further neurological injury; therefore, diagnostics such as ventrodorsal radiographs and abdominal ultrasound should be avoided until the disease causing the neurological deficits is defined. Serology and polymerase chain reaction (PCR) tests for infectious disease may be done at the time of a minimum database if they are indicated based on clinical suspicion.

Diagnostic plan for rabbits with brain disease

Once a rabbit's neurological deficits are localized to a specific area of the brain, a list of possible causes should be formulated. To evaluate the brain, advanced imaging such as CT or MRI may be done. MRI is preferred for evaluation of soft tissue, such as the brain. Readers can refer to the article by Marguerite F. Knipe in this issue for further details regarding imaging techniques. General anesthesia is required in rabbits for both CT and

MRI. Anesthetic agents that increase intracranial pressure should be avoided. MRI generally requires prolonged anesthesia, and because of the magnetic field of the equipment, specialized anesthetic equipment is required. CSF sampling, for microbiologic and cytologic analyses, generally is done following MRI or CT. CSF should be collected caudal to the lesion, and therefore in rabbits with brain disease, CSF is collected from the cisterna magna. Electrophysiological tests such as a brainstem auditory evoked response (BAER) (for vestibulocochlear problems) and electroencephalogram (EEG) (for seizure disorders) may be indicated in some rabbits.

Diagnostic plan for rabbits with spinal cord disease

Many spinal cord conditions may be diagnosed using noncontrast radiographic procedures (ideally with the rabbit under general anesthesia). Examples include vertebral fractures/luxations (Fig. 12), congenital vertebral anomalies, vertebral neoplasia, and infectious conditions such as discospondylitis. CSF analysis may be useful in further categorizing the disease process, or in some instances, making a definitive diagnosis. CSF is collected under anesthesia by cisternal or lumbar subarachnoid puncture. CSF abnormalities are more likely to be found if the sample is collected close to the lesion. CSF should be collected before myelography, because contrast agents may alter CSF parameters [8].

Myelography

Injection of contrast material into the subarachnoid space to outline of the spinal cord is indicated when noncontrast radiography and CSF analysis fail to fully define the cause of a myelopathy, or when a precise localization for spinal surgery is needed. Lumbar injection of contrast material is preferred. Use of oblique views and dynamic projections may maximize

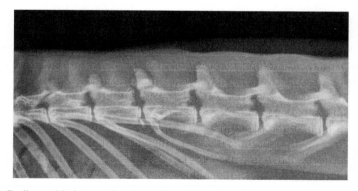

Fig. 12. Radiographic image of a domestic rabbit (*Oryctolagus cuniculus*) in lateral recumbency. This rabbit had a history of trauma and resultant paraplegia. Note the fracture/luxation of T13-L1 articular facets and endplate of T13.

diagnostic information. Readers can refer to the article by Marguerite F. Knipe in this issue for more details.

MRI and CT

MRI and CT are less invasive than myelography. Additionally, they allow for transverse images of the spinal cord to be viewed and provide better definition of spinal cord parenchyma and surrounding structures. CT generally is done following myelography to further define a focal lesion. Although MRI is preferred for imaging soft tissues such as the spinal cord, resolution of spinal cord lesions in small rabbits may be problematic, and it may be difficult to obtain complete surveys of the spinal cord. Accessibility to imaging facilities and the high cost of imaging procedures are major considerations in rabbits.

Diagnosis of neuromuscular disease

After the minimum database is completed, the next diagnostic steps for rabbits with neuromuscular disease are electrophysiology (electromyography, nerve conduction velocity testing), and nerve and/or muscle biopsy.

Summary

Companion rabbits commonly are presented to veterinary practitioners for assessment of neurological signs. Neurologic disease in rabbits is common because of the incidence of several infectious diseases and the potential for traumatic injury in this species. Despite the paucity of scientific literature regarding the neuroanatomy of this common laboratory animal, the minimal information that does exist for rabbits can be combined with basic concepts from canine species and applied to examine rabbits neurologically and localize lesions in rabbits. The information provided in this article helps to establish guidelines for performing a neurological examination in a rabbit, but the temperament of each animal must be assessed carefully to avoid inadvertent traumatic lesions of the spinal cord.

Further readings

Garosi L. The neurological examination. In: Platt SR, Olby NJ, editors. BSAVA manual of canine and feline neurology. Gloucester (UK): British Small Animal Veterinary Association; 2004. p. 1–23.
Lorenz MD, Kornegay JN. Neurologic history and examination. In: Lorenz MD, Kornegay JN, editors. Handbook of veterinary neurology. St. Louis (MO): Sanders; 2004. p. 1–44.

References

[1] Wingerd B, Stein G. Rabbit dissection manual. 1st edition. Baltimore (MD): The Johns Hopkins University Press; 1985.

[2] Harcourt-Brown F. Textbook of rabbit medicine. Oxford (UK): Butterworth Heinemann; 2002.

[3] Greenaway J, Partlow G, Gonsholt N, et al. Anatomy of the lumbosacral spinal cord in rabbits. J Am Anim Hosp Assoc 2001;37:27–34.

[4] McLaughlin C, Chiasson R. Laboratory anatomy of the rabbit. 2nd edition. Dubuque (IA): William C Brown; 1979.

[5] Evans H. Miller's anatomy of the dog. 3rd edition. Philadelphia: WB Saunders Co; 1993.

[6] Biricik HS, Oguz H, Sindak N, et al. Evaluation of the Schirmer and phenol red thread tests for measuring tear secretion in rabbits. Vet Rec 2005;156(15):485–7.

[7] King AS. Physiological and clinical anatomy of the domestic mammals, vol. I. London (UK): Blackwell Science; 1987.

[8] Burbidge HM, Kannegieter N, Dickson LR, et al. Iohexol myelography in the horse. Equine Vet J 1989;21(5):347–50.

ELSEVIER
SAUNDERS

VETERINARY
CLINICS
Exotic Animal Practice

Vet Clin Exot Anim 10 (2007) 759–773

Clinical Neurology of Ferrets

Orlando Diaz-Figueroa, DVM, MS,
DABVP (Avian)[a],*, Mary O. Smith, BVM&S, PhD,
DACVIM (Neurology)[b]

[a]Lake Howell Animal Clinic, 856 Lake Howell Rd, Maitland, FL 32751, USA
[b]9905 South U.S. Highway 17-92, Maitland, FL 32751, USA

Neurological diseases often are encountered in pet ferrets (*Mustela putorius furo*). The most common presenting complaint is paraparesis/paralysis and ataxia. Primary neurologic diseases, however, are not common in pet ferrets. Clinical presentations caused by primary neurologic disease are a frequent manifestation of systemic illness. The principal causes of neurological disease in ferrets include bacterial, fungal, viral, parasitic, neoplastic, traumatic lesions, and congenital anomalies. Accurate case assessment and diagnosis of neurological problems in this species can be challenging for the veterinary practitioner. The increased availability of advanced diagnostic imaging techniques, such as CT and MRI, however, has made obtaining a final diagnosis a more attainable goal. This article discusses the more common neurological disorders of ferrets, including the various diagnostic procedures that can be used to investigate them, and treatment options available.

The nervous system often is thought of as the bodily system that is least accessible for examination. The reality, however, is that the functioning of the nervous system can be observed in every movement, action, and reaction of an animal, and the presence of disease within the nervous system usually is readily discernible by observation of the patient. Recognition and diagnosis of neurological disease depends on knowledge of normal behaviors and reactions of a species, so that the abnormal can be detected. Neurological examination is the foundation of clinical neurology, because it allows the clinician to answer the questions "Is neurological disease present?" and "Where is the location of the disease along the neuroaxis?" Localization narrows the differential diagnosis list and dictates the most appropriate

* Corresponding author.
E-mail address: dr.diaz@lakehowellanimalclinic.com (O. Diaz-Figueroa).

diagnostic tests. Fortunately for the veterinarian, the nervous systems of all mammals are remarkably alike. Studies of the ferret brain have revealed that its general structure and functional organization resemble that of other carnivores, particularly the cat among the domesticated species [1,2]. Techniques for neurological examination of species such as cats and dogs are applicable to ferrets, and interpretation of the findings is broadly similar. Most of the categories of neurological disease that occur in other species (eg, trauma, neoplasia, infection) also have been described in the ferret, and many specific disease entities are the same (eg, rabies virus infection). On the other hand, some diseases have a particular prevalence in this species (eg, Aleutian disease and chordomas).

Neurological examination and diagnostics

Evaluation of any animal with suspected neurological disease always must begin with a thorough physical examination. Systemic diseases and diseases of organs such as the liver and pancreas may cause secondary involvement of the nervous system (eg, hepatic encephalopathy, or hypoglycemia because of an insulin-secreting tumor). Additionally, any systemic illness in a ferret may result in weakness that mimics primary neurological disease. Overall observation, assessment of rectal temperature, pulse and respiratory rates, auscultation of the heart and lungs, evaluation of mucous membranes, and palpation of the abdomen and lymph nodes usually are performed before neurological examination. An alternative system of examination is to perform the examination from nose to tail, evaluating all organ systems in each region of the body. Orthopedic examination should be performed to help differentiate neurological and musculoskeletal causes of paresis and abnormal gait.

The neurological examination in ferrets is similar to that for other domestic animal species. Ferrets are usually fairly amenable to handling, which facilitates neurological examination. Specific details of examination techniques and localization of neurological lesions will not be covered in this article, but many texts describe the neurological examination of cats and dogs in detail, and these techniques are generally applicable to ferrets [3–5]. Similarly, principles of localization of neurological lesions in other domestic animal species also apply to the ferret. Examination should commence with observation of the patient at a distance. The level and appropriateness of consciousness are evaluated; then posture and gait are observed with attention to strength and symmetry. When the animal is examined outside its usual environment, some allowances should be made for the effects of stress and fear, which often may alter normal responses. Cranial nerve assessment is similar to that of other small mammals; pupillary light reflexes, facial sensation, facial symmetry, tongue movement, and swallowing are assessed easily. Ferrets have darkly pigmented irises and hidden sclera; therefore vestibular eye movements are difficult to evaluate. Many normal ferrets lack a consistent menace response. The vestibular system should be assessed by checking for resting or positional nystagmus or strabismus, head tilt, and leaning or falling to one side. Conscious proprioception is evaluated by testing hopping and placing reactions. Myotactic (tendon) reflexes should be evaluated using the handle of a hemostat or similar instrument to percuss the patellar and tricep tendons. The accurate evaluation of myotactic reflexes in ferrets is somewhat limited by their small size and short limbs. Limb withdrawal strength and conscious pain perception should be evaluated by lightly pinching between or across the digits of each foot using a hemostat or similar instrument just strongly enough to elicit both reflex flexion and a conscious response to the stimulus. Note that ferrets with diverse metabolic disorders or other systemic illnesses may present with posterior paresis, giving the false impression of a myelopathy. To further complicate matters, these ferrets may have questionable posterior proprioceptive positioning.

Tests applicable to the diagnosis of neurological disease in ferrets are, broadly speaking, similar to those commonly used in the cat and dog. Serum biochemistry, complete blood count, and urinalysis are required to help rule out some of the systemic diseases that can cause weakness in ferrets that can mimic myelopathy. Hypoglycemia caused by insulin-secreting tumor also is an important differential diagnosis for many neurological diseases in this species. Radiographic studies of the vertebral column and skull can reveal evidence of traumatic, lytic, proliferative, and neoplastic lesions involving bone. Myelography aids in the diagnosis of compressive and expansile lesions affecting the spinal cord. The use of CT and MRI has been reported in ferrets and adds invaluable information for diagnosis of both intracranial and spinal lesions. Doses for contrast agents for use with each of these modalities have been reported previously [6]. For CT, iothalamate sodium (Conray 400, 2.2 mL/kg of 400 mg/mL) has been reported to be used as a contrast agent, and for MRI, gadolinium diethylenetriamine pentaacetic acid (Gd-DTPA, 0.2 mL/kg) has been used.

Cerebrospinal fluid analysis (CSF) is particularly helpful in the diagnosis of infectious diseases of the central nervous system (CNS). CSF is obtained most easily in ferrets from the cisterna magna. Briefly, after clipping the skin over the atlanto–occipital region the skin is surgically prepared with a sterile scrub. With the head of the patient flexed at a right angle (90 degrees) to the long axis of the body, a 25 gauge, 1.6 cm long hypodermic needle is used to gently puncture the skin and enter the cisterna magna, and the CSF is allowed to drip into a collection tube. Reference ranges for CSF in the ferret have been reported and are provided in Table 1. Blood contamination of CSF during the tap procedure is fairly common; this has minimal effect on the protein concentration of CSF, but may cause a significantly false elevation in the nucleated cell content. CSF also may be collected from the lumbar subarachnoid space. Reference values for lumbar CSF from ferrets have not been published, but protein concentration may be expected

Table 1
Reference ranges and mean values for constituents of cerebrospinal fluid collected from the
cisterna magna of healthy ferrets

Parameter	Reference range	Mean
Nucleated cells per μL	0.00–8.00	1.59
Total protein μg/μL	28.00–68.00	31.40

(*Data from* Platt SR, Dennis PM, McSherry LJ, et al: Composition of cerebrospinal fluid in
clinically normal adult ferrets. Am J Vet Res 2004;65:758–60.)

to be slightly higher than for cisternal CSF, similar to what has been found
in other species.

Common domestic ferret diseases with neurologic signs

The following discussion is meant to serve as an overall review of diseases
that affect ferrets and can cause them to present with neurological signs. In
some cases, the diseases are described in their entirety (not just focusing on
the neurologic system) to allow practitioners to gain a better understanding
of clinical presentation, diagnosis, and pathology. The diseases mentioned
are included, because they are common, have been minimally described elsewhere, or are diseases of clinical importance.

Bacterial diseases

Clostridium botulinum

Ferrets are moderately susceptible to botulism (*Clostridium botulinum*)
types A and B, and they are highly susceptible to botulism type C [7–13].
In Europe, botulism has killed animals in fur farms and occasionally
hunting ferrets. Fortunately, the *Clostridium* bacteria are typically susceptible to antibiotics, but the effect of the endotoxin produced by the organism
on the nervous system is rapid. The ferret, like mink, is less resistant to the
endotoxin effects than is the dog or other carnivores [10]. Clinical signs
including dysphagia, ataxia, and paresis appear 12 to 96 hours after eating
contaminated foods [11–13]. Respiration is shallow because of partial
paralysis of the intercostal muscles and diaphragm. Salivation and protrusion of the third eyelid occur, and finally death results from respiratory
failure.

Although a presumptive diagnosis of a clostridial infection is based on
clinical signs of flaccid paralysis, definitive diagnosis requires demonstration
of the presence of botulinum toxin in food or clinical specimens such as
blood, serum, or gastrointestinal (GI) contents [7–10]. Both in vivo and in
vitro tests are available for identification of botulinum toxin. The most
common in vivo test is the neutralization test in mice. In vitro tests include
radioimmunoassay and enzyme-linked immunosorbent assay (ELISA);
however, these tests usually are not sufficient alone, because of their

predilection to measure the antigenicity rather than the toxigenicity of the toxin produced [14]. Treatment consists of administration of type C antitoxin and supportive care. A bacterin for the *C. botulinum* type C is available for immunization of mink and ferrets being fed fresh meat diets [12,13].

Viral diseases

Canine distemper

One of the most common and devastating infectious diseases affecting the domestic ferret is canine distemper virus (CDV). Distemper virus was first described by Dunkin and Laidlaw in 1926 during their initial investigation of distemper virus in dogs [15]. Because of its extreme susceptibility to the disease, the ferret has been used widely since then to characterize the disease in the dog and was instrumental in the development of effective vaccines for use in dogs. Canine distemper virus is a member of the *Paramyxoviridae* family and is related closely to rinderpest and measles viruses. The virus is susceptible to ultraviolet light, heat, and drying conditions, and survives outside the host only for short periods. Commonly used disinfectants are effective in destroying the virus [16]. The natural hosts of canine distemper virus include many species of terrestrial carnivores, including Ailuridae (lesser panda), Canidae (dog, dingo, fox, coyote, jackal, wolf), Hyaenidae (hyena), Procyonidae (raccoon, kinkajou, coati, bassariscus), Viverridae (binturong), Mustelidae (weasel, ferret, mink, skunk, badger, otter, stoat, marten), and possibly some members of Felidae [17,18]. Species within the Mustelidae family, including domestic ferret and mink, are considered to be among the most susceptible to infection by canine distemper virus and to its pathogenic effects.

Epizootiology

Transmission of canine distemper virus to ferrets occurs by contact with infected dogs, ferrets, or (theoretically) wild carnivores. The virus is shed in the nasal exudate and saliva of infected animals and readily spread by aerosolization of the virus particles [19]. Excretion of virus by ferrets begins in the fifth day after inoculation, and viral shedding continues until the death of the animal [19]. Once the infection has been established in a susceptible colony, it is probable that the entire stock will be affected. Immunity to infection is of long duration, probably lifelong. Because recovery from natural infection is exceedingly unusual, however, immune animals rarely are encountered. For the same reason, recovered carrier animals are not a significant source of infection for other ferrets [19,20].

Pathogenesis

Naturally acquired infection in ferrets follows an initial course similar to that in dogs. Two days after aerosol exposure through the upper respiratory tract, viral replication occurs in the regional lymph nodes of the respiratory tract. The virus quickly spreads to the mediastinal and mesenteric lymph nodes, spleen, Kupffer's cells of the liver, and the leukocytes of the peripheral blood. Viremia occurs on the fourth or fifth day after exposure, as evidenced by the presence of viral antigen in mononuclear cells [19]. After approximately 1 week, further hematogenous spread of the virus occurs, affecting the epithelium of the respiratory tract, GI tract, cutaneous tissues, urinary tract, and superficial ocular tissue.

The respiratory tract, along with lymphoid tissue, is a major site for viral replication, with antigen concentration reaching a maximum on day 12 after inoculation [19,21,22]. Viral antigen persists in the infected tissues until the death of the animal. CNS invasion and replication also can occur. In the ferret (as in the dog), certain strains of the virus are neurotrophic, and CNS infection is seen more commonly [19–22]. Secondary bacterial infection of the respiratory, GI, cutaneous, or superficial ocular tissues may complicate the disease process.

Clinical findings

Clinical signs of distemper in the ferret reflect the fact that the virus is pantrophic (capable of replicating in a wide variety of cells) [19,21,22]. Unlike in the dog, however, the course of the disease is fairly constant, with a predictable progression of findings. The incubation period usually ranges from 4 to 10 days, with the onset of clinical signs typically occurring 7 to 9 days after exposure. Consistent findings during this period include anorexia, fever, and a mucopurulent conjunctivitis. The ocular discharge is often the first sign noted, and the eyelids may stick together with dry, purulent crusts. Additional ocular findings can include severe blepharitis, keratoconjunctivitis sicca, and corneal ulceration [19]. Several days after the ocular signs are evident, erythematous cutaneous rashes develop in the inguinal area, beneath the chin, and on the foot pads. Hyperkeratosis of the foot pads is highly suggestive of distemper virus [19]. Clinical findings related to the respiratory tract vary from catarrhal rhinitis to severe, fulminating pneumonia, often complicated by secondary bacterial pathogens. GI infection is evidenced by loose stools and diarrhea, which may be dark and tarry. Animals surviving the acute catarrhal phase may develop CNS infection with associated myoclonus, paresis, muscular tremors, hyperexcitability, convulsions, or coma [20–23].

Ferrets usually succumb to the effect of the disease within 1 week from the onset of clinical signs; however, this time interval varies with the virus strain. Death has been reported as soon as 2 days and as late as 35 days after inoculation [19,21,23]. The mortality associated with distemper is believed to be related to several factors, most notably widespread replication and necrosis in lymphoid tissue and circulating lymphocytes with associated immunosuppression.

Diagnosis

Clinical signs of distemper are highly suggestive of the disease; however, other viral infections of the ferret, most notably human influenza virus infection, produce a nasal and ocular discharge that might be confused with distemper. For this reason, and because canine distemper virus has such significant implications for pet owners or research colonies, prompt diagnosis is required.

Rapid antemortem diagnosis is usually possible through the use of fluorescent antibody techniques on a blood smear, buffy coat preparation, or conjunctival scraping [19]. Despite the fact that less than 1% of the circulating leukocytes contain viral antigen, mononuclear cell fluorescence is found 2 to 3 days after experimental inoculation and is invariably positive by the sixth day [19]. Conjunctival epithelial fluorescence occurs slightly later, usually becoming positive by the ninth day of infection. Conjunctival epithelium and leukocytes are reported to continue to exhibit a positive fluorescence throughout the course of the disease [24]. False-negative results may be encountered if leucopenia is present. Serum antibody levels to canine distemper virus can aid in diagnosis [19,24,25]. In experimentally-infected ferrets, a reverse transcriptase-polymerase chain reaction (RT-PCR) has been used to detect the virus in peripheral blood. Recently, nested PCR was found to be a sensitive and specific method for diagnosis of CDV infection [10,19,25].

Postmortem diagnosis is usually straight forward, because widespread distemper inclusions are present in tissues. Viral isolation, although time-consuming, is an additional means of confirming infection. Intraperitoneal administration of suspension of spleen, liver, or lung of infected ferrets to tests ferrets, results in typical signs and course of the disease [10]. The virus also can be isolated in vitro on canine lung macrophages or ferret kidney cells, both of which exhibit characteristic cytopathic effects when infected [21].

Pathologic findings

Gross pathologic findings often are limited to the cutaneous and ocular abnormalities noted on physical examination. A catarrhal and/or hemorrhagic tracheitis or bronchitis may be present [19,21]. Inclusion bodies are the most remarkable diagnostic feature on histopathologic examination. Distemper virus inclusions are eosinophilic or acidophilic rounded structures more commonly found in the cytoplasm but also present in nuclei. They represent viral particles and cellular components associated with the virus. Inclusions are identified easily in the epithelium of the bronchi, renal pelvis, urinary bladder, stomach, biliary ducts, and conjunctiva. Inclusion are present but less numerous in the skin epithelium, hair follicles, reticulum cells of the spleen, small intestinal epithelium, corneal epithelium, and glia and neurons of the CNS. Hyperkeratosis and parakeratosis of the epidermis (including the foot pads), hair follicles, and sebaceous glands often are identified [10,19]. Reports of pathologic findings in the CNS are limited because of the acute fulminating nature of the disease. Scattered neuronal degeneration has been described with CNS infection [19–26].

Therapy and prevention

Because of the high mortality associated with CDV in ferrets, euthanasia has been suggested as an acceptable alternative to symptomatic care [10,19,20]. Should therapy be attempted for pet ferrets, it should be entirely supportive and should include maintenance of hydration with subcutaneous fluids, parenteral bactericidal antibiotics, and topical antibacterial ophthalmic ointments. Thorough daily disinfection of the environment is indicated. The virus is inactivated by heat, visible light, and commonly used disinfectants (ie, 0.2% roccal, 2% sodium hydroxide, and 0.1% formalin). Some researchers reported that out of 1000 cases of canine distemper, not a single ferret survived the infection [10,19,20].

Vaccination against CDV with attenuated live virus strains is the only effective means by which to prevent the disease in susceptible ferrets or to control the disease during an outbreak. One vaccine is approved for use in ferrets in North America. Purevax Ferret Distemper Vaccine (Merial, Athens, Georgia) is a lyophilized vaccine of a recombinant canary pox vector that expresses the HA and F glycoprotein of CDV [26]. The absence of adjuvant decreases the risk of adverse reactions. The manufacturer reported an incidence of anaphylactic reactions of 0.3% in its field safety trials [26]. Another modified-live canine distemper vaccine attenuated in primate cell line (Galaxy D, Schering Plough Animal Health, Omaha, Nebraska) has been used in ferrets. This vaccine was effective in preventing canine distemper in young ferrets; however, the duration of immunity and the incidence of vaccine reaction are unknown. Galaxy D is extra label (not approved for use in ferrets by US Department of Agriculture [USDA]) and requires informed consent from the owner. Therefore, vaccination of ferrets with these products is not recommended.

Aleutian disease

Aleutian disease virus (ADV) is a parvovirus that causes persistent infection in mink [6,27]. The only animal besides mink in which overt disease appears to occur is the ferret. Diagnosis of ADV in ferrets is based on the same criteria as for mink. ADV in ferrets is characterized by an illness with chronic wasting, hypergammaglobulinemia and a high serum antibody titer to ADV, plasmacytic–lymphocytic infiltration in multiple organs, dilation and proliferation of the bile ducts, and global membranous glomerulopathy and vasculitis [6,27,28]. Characteristic clinical signs in ferrets with ADV infection include splenic enlargement, lymphadenopathy, pelvic limb ataxia, paraparesis, or quadriplegia [6,27]. Paraplegia accompanied by urinary and fecal incontinence occurs occasionally. Differential diagnoses for paraplegia caused by ADV include CDV infection, rabies, fungal or mycobacterial infection, intervertebral disc disease, vertebral fractures, tumors of the spinal cord, and hematomyelia associated with estrus-induced anemia [29]. ADV is shed in feces and urine and can be transmitted horizontally by the oral route. Infection also can occur with exposure to fomites, and in a vertical manner from dam to kits [6,27,29].

In the ferret, ADV infection causes a disseminated nonsuppurative encephalomyelitis [30]. Other histopathologic lesions of the disease include peri-vascular accumulation of mononuclear cells, astrocyte hypertrophy, and parenchymal vacuolation of the meninges suggestive of demyelination [30]. Veterinary practitioners should submit serum for ADV antibody testing by counterimmunoelectrophoresis (United Vaccines, Madison, Wisconsin) or ELISA (Avecon Diagnostics, Bath, Pennsylvania) [6]. Clinically normal ferrets with positive titers do not necessarily develop clinical signs. There is no treatment [20]. Affected ferrets should be isolated or euthanized to decrease the spread of the virus. ADV probably persists in infected ferrets for years. There is no cross-antigenicity between ADV and other parvovirus vaccines, and there is no specific vaccine because of the immune-mediated nature of the disease [27].

Rabies

There have been several cases of rabies reported in ferrets in the United States [19]. Clinical signs include lethargy, anxiety, paresthesia, posterior paresis, and other signs of CNS disease [19]. The virus has been detected in the salivary glands and in saliva of rabid ferrets [31]. A killed vaccine has been approved for yearly use in ferrets (Imrab 3, Rhone Merieux, Athens, Georgia), but it may not be considered protective if the vaccinated animal bites a human. Owing to governmental regulations, even ferrets vaccinated against rabies virus may still need to be sacrificed if it has bitten a human. Inform ferret owners at the time of vaccination of any local or state laws that may apply.

Neoplasia

Neoplasia affecting the nervous system has been reported uncommonly in ferrets, despite this species' apparent susceptibility to neoplasia in other organs [32,33]. As with all diseases of the nervous system, the signs associated with neoplasia depend on its location within the nervous system, not the specific tumor type. Although signs may be slowly progressive in some cases, in others, the onset of signs may be acute and the progression of disease rapid. Similar findings have been described in many other species.

Lymphoma

T cell lymphoma limited to the spine has been described in a 22-month-old ferret [34]. The ferret presented with acute onset of paraparesis that progressed within hours to paralysis and incontinence. Radiographs and CT scan revealed a soft tissue mass and associated lysis of a lumbar vertebra. Diagnosis was made on the basis of cytology of a fine needle aspirate from the mass, and eventual necropsy. There were several unique features of the lymphoma in this patient compared with most ferrets with T cell lymphoma. The animal was slightly older then the typical ferret with lymphoma (usually under 1 year old). The signs were peracute and very rapidly progressive. There was a complete lack of response to prednisone therapy. No other organs were involved; in particular, there was no lymphocytosis, lymphadenopathy, splenomegaly, or mediastinal mass [35]. The significance of the unique features of the lymphoma in this patient is unknown.

Chordoma

Chordomas are rare neoplasms of the spinal cord in most species, but they have been reported quite frequently in the ferret [32,36]. They are thought to develop from the remnants of the embryonic notochord. Most chordomas in ferrets appear as firm, slowly-growing, multilobulated masses in the tails of mature adults; they may ulcerate [37–39]. Most develop toward or at the distal extremity of the tail. A higher incidence in females is suspected [36]. Cytology of fine needle aspirates from these tumors may be diagnostic; the use of immunohistochemical stains for proteins such as vimentin, cytokeratin, S-100, and others facilitates diagnosis and aids differentiation from chondrosarcomas, which are histologically similar [36,37,40,41]. Treatment is by amputation of the tail proximal to the tumor, leaving a wide tissue margin. Prognosis after surgery is usually good when the tumor is located distally. Extensive metastasis has been reported, however, after removal of a chordoma located near the base of the tail [42]. In this case, the tumor had been present for 4 years before excision, a factor that may have contributed to the widespread metastases.

Chordomas occur occasionally in regions of the spine other than the tail, where they can cause more severe clinical signs and are treated less easily. The clinical signs described with chordomas affecting the thoracic and cervical regions of the spine are as expected for any focal myelopathy: progressive paresis and loss of proprioception caudal to the tumor, which may progress to paralysis [41,43]. Animals may become incontinent of both feces and urine, and lose the ability to voluntarily empty the bladder. The signs are caused by increasing compression of the spinal cord by the expanding tumor. Surgical excision has been performed, but outcomes have been poor because of several factors: severity of clinical signs by the time of diagnosis, local recurrence, and (rarely) metastasis, especially to the skin [41,43].

Other spinal tumors

Plasma cell myeloma has been reported in an adult ferret that had progressive paraparesis over 8 months, terminating in paraplegia with loss of pain perception caudal to the lesion. The tumor was found at necropsy; it had eroded the vertebral body of L6, resulting in pathological fracture with subsequent myelomalacia. Unfortunately, this tumor was diagnosed only at necropsy, so clinical data such as radiographic and serum biochemical findings were not available. It seems reasonable to hypothesize, however, that features common in other species with plasma cell tumors, such as radiographic evidence of lytic bone lesions and the presence of monoclonal gammopathy also may be found in ferrets. Efficacy of medical therapy for plasma cell tumors is unknown in the ferret.

Skull and brain tumors

Osteoma arising from the skull has been described in ferrets [44,45]. Osteomas are benign tumors of bone that cause clinical signs when they impinge on surrounding tissues. In one of the cases reported, the signs occurred when the osteoma, which appeared to have arisen from the temporal or occipital bone, impinged on the airways (larynx, trachea) resulting in respiratory distress. Signs caused by compression of the brain can include mental dullness, paresis, and proprioceptive deficits. Other signs such as circling and seizures could be expected, depending on the location of the tumor. These tumors are often large before they cause clinical signs, and frequently they are observable or palpable externally. Radiographic or CT imaging facilitates diagnosis [46]. Surgical excision may be possible.

A granular cell tumor affecting the brain (myoblastoma) has been reported in the ferret [47]. Clinical signs may be chronic to subacute to acute in onset, and reflect the region of the brain involved. Seizures are a common finding, but head tilt, circling, ataxia, paresis, disorientation, and mental dullness all may occur. Neck pain is a well-recognized manifestation of some intracranial tumors in other species, such as dogs, and this has been described in the ferret [47]. In animals where a brain tumor is suspected, modalities such as CT and magnetic resonance scans are appropriate for diagnosis. Differential diagnoses are legion, including all the various infectious, toxic, and metabolic causes of brain dysfunction discussed elsewhere in this article.

Intervertebral disc herniation

Herniation of thoracolumbar intervertebral discs has been reported several times in ferrets [48–50]. Ferrets presented with signs of acute myelopathy: loss of proprioception and paresis to paralysis caudal to the lesion. Diagnosis was made by means of noncontrast radiographs or myelography. A narrowed intervertebral disc space was observed on radiographs in one case, while myelography revealed an extradural mass in another. In the latter case, subluxation of the vertebrae on either side of the herniated disc also was present; the signs in this animal were of several months duration, and the exact relationship between the subluxation and the disc herniation was unclear. Other diagnostic modalities such as CT and MRI are extremely helpful for diagnosing disc herniation in dogs and cats, and should also be useful in ferrets, when they are available. Although conservative treatment with a corticosteroid (prednisone, 5 mg once daily) and rest resulted in resolution of signs in one ferret [48], surgical decompression is the therapeutic modality that most directly addresses the disease process. Surgical decompression of the spinal cord by means of hemilaminectomy has been performed successfully in ferrets with disc herniations, and prognosis is likely to be good as long as pain perception is still present caudal to the lesion when the patient is presented for surgery [49,50]. Information on long term prognosis and the possibility of recurrence of disc herniation at other sites is not yet available.

Miscellaneous diseases

Pregnant and postparturient females are predisposed to several nutrition-dependent diseases, such as eclampsia toxemia and nursing sickness. Although hypocalcemia, hypophosphatemia, and ketosis may develop, neurologic signs are rare unless hepatic lipidosis is so severe that encephalopathy is present [6].

Posterior paralysis accompanied by incontinence may appear in an otherwise healthy animal. This paralysis may be caused by hemivertebrae, vertebral fractures, intervertebral disk disease, hematomyelia, or myelitis.

Ferrets are subject to various spontaneous and congenital neurological malformations that may be hereditary. These include anencephaly, neuroschisis, and amyelia. A report of copper toxicosis in two ferrets was believed to be congenital. Iniencephaly also has been reported in ferrets [51,52].

CNS depression and lethargy because of systemic mycoses have been reported in ferrets [6,10,21]. *Cryptococcus* species have been identified as a cause of meningitis in ferrets [6,11]. Systemic blastomycosis also has been identified in ferrets, with multifocal granulomatous meningoencephalitis [6,11]. Diagnoses of these diseases have been through clinical signs, radiographic changes, and isolation of the causative organism. Impression smears of draining tracts or CSF may be useful in identifying the organism.

All carnivores are susceptible to toxoplasmosis and the ferret possibly could act as an intermediate host to *Toxoplasma gondii*. Toxoplasmosis has been identified in ferrets, and clinical signs most likely have developed secondary to exposure to cat feces and raw meat [53,54]. *Toxoplasma gondii* has been found, on histology, in experimental ferrets used for distemper research and also has been obtained in three ferrets by means of in vivo passage of brain tissue in mice [53,54].

Summary

Primary neurological disorders are not common in pet ferrets. As ferrets are anatomically and physiologically similar to dogs and cats, the basic elements of ferret neurological examination, disease processes, and preventive health are familiar to the small-animal practitioner. These characteristics make ferrets amenable to many of the highly specialized diagnostics and therapeutics that are now available in small animal practice. Veterinarians should not forget to draw from the wealth of knowledge in canine and feline medicine when managing unusual or difficult disorders in ferret patients.

References

[1] Lockard BI. The forebrain of the ferret. Lab Anim Sci 1985;35:216–28.
[2] Lawes INC, Andrews PLR. Neuroanatomy of the ferret brain. In: Fox JG, editor. Biology and diseases of the ferret. 2nd edition. Baltimore (MD): Lippincott Williams & Wilkins; 1998. p. 71–102.
[3] Smith MO. Neurological examination for the busy practitioner. Denver (CO): AAHA Press; 2002.
[4] Oliver JE Jr, Lorenz MD, Kornegay JN. Handbook of veterinary neurology. 3rd edition. Philadelphia: W.B. Saunders; 1997. p. 3–46.
[5] Bagley RS. Fundamentals of veterinary clinical neurology. Ames (IA): Blackwell Publishing; 2005. p. 57–108.
[6] Antinoff N. Musculoskeletal and neurological diseases. In: Quesenberry KE, Carpenter JW, editors. Ferrets, rabbits and rodents: clinical medicine and surgery. 2nd edition. Philadelphia: W.B. Saunders; 1997. p. 115–20.
[7] Ryland LM, Gorham JR. The ferret and its diseases. J Am Vet Med Assoc 1978;173: 1154–8.
[8] Andrews PL, Illman O, Mellersh A. Some observation of anatomical abnormalities and disease states in a population of 350 ferrets (Mustela furo L). Z Versuchstierkd 1979;21: 346–53.
[9] Anon N. Husbandry and diseases of mink management. In: The Merck veterinary manual. 7th edition. Rahway (NJ); 1991. p. 1050–6.
[10] Lewington JH. Viral, bacterial and mycotic diseases. In: Lewington JH, editor. Ferret husbandry, medicine, and surgery. 1st edition. Woburn (MA): Butterworth Heinemann; 2000. p. 106–28.
[11] Fox JG. Mycotic diseases. In: Fox JG, editor. Biology and diseases of the ferret. 2nd edition. Baltimore (MD): Lippincott Williams and Wilkins; 1998. p. 393–403.
[12] Quartrup ER, Gorham JR. Susceptible of fur-bearing animals to toxins of C. botulinum types A, B, C, and E. Am J Vet Res 1949;10:268.
[13] Harrison SG, Borland ED. Deaths in Ferrets (Mustela putorius) due to Clostridium botulinum type C. Vet Rec 1973;93:576.
[14] Greene CE, editor. Infectious disease of the dog and cat. 2nd edition. Philadelphia: W.B. Saunders; 1990. p. 763–78.
[15] Dunkin GW, Laidlaw PP. Studies in dog distemper: I. Dog distemper in the ferret. J Comp Pathol Ther 1926;39:201–12.
[16] Greene CE. Canine distemper. In: Greene CE, editor. Clinical microbiology and infectious diseases of the dog and cat. Philadelphia: W.B. Saunders; 1984. p. 386–406.
[17] Keymer IF, Epps HBG. Canine Distemper in the family Mustelidae. Vet Rec 1969;85(7): 204–5.
[18] Bush M, Montali RJ, Browstein D, et al. Vaccine-induced canine distemper in a lesser panda. J Am Vet Med Assoc 1976;169(9):959–60.
[19] Fox JG, Pearson RC, Gorham JR. Viral and chlamydial diseases. In: Fox JG, editor. Biology and diseases of Ferrets. Philadelphia: Lea & Febiger; 1988. p. 186–96.

[20] Besch –Williford CL. Biology and medicine of the ferret. Vet Clinic North Am Small Anim Pract 1987;17:1155–83.
[21] Crook E, Mcnutt SH. Experimental distemper in mink and ferrets. II. Appearance and significance of histopathologic changes. Am J Vet Res 1959;20(75):378–83.
[22] Larin NM. Canine distemper virus in the ferret. J Comp Pathol Ther 1955;65:325–33.
[23] Kilham L, Haberman RT, Herman CM. Jaundice and bilirubinemia as manifestation of canine distemper in raccoons and ferrets. Am J Vet Res 1956;17(62):144–8.
[24] Lui C, Coffin DL. Studies on canine distemper infection by means of fluorescein-labeled antibody. I. The pathogenesis, pathology, and diagnosis of disease in experimentally infected ferrets. Virology 1957;3:115–31.
[25] Kauffman CA, Bergman AG, O'Connor RP. Distemper virus infection in ferrets: an animal model of measles-induced immunosuppression. Clin Exp Immunol 1982;47:617–25.
[26] Langlois I. Viral diseases of ferrets. Vet Clin North Am Exot Anim Pract 2005;8(1):139–60.
[27] Welchman DdeB, Oxenham M, Done SH. Aleutian disease in domestic ferrets: diagnostic findings and survey results. Vet Rec 1993;132:479–84.
[28] Rozengurt N, Stewart S, Sanchez S. Diagnostic exercise: ataxia and incoordination in ferrets. Lab Anim Sci 1995;45:432–4.
[29] Fox JG. Systemic diseases. In: Fox JG, editor. Biology and diseases of ferrets. Philadelphia: Lea & Febiger; 1988. p. 255–73.
[30] Palley LS, Corning BF, Fox JG, et al. Parvovirus-associated syndrome (Aleutian disease) in two ferrets. J Am Vet Med Assoc 1992;201(1):100–6.
[31] Niezgoda M, Briggs DJ, Shaddock J, et al. Viral excretion in domestic ferrets... inoculated with a raccoon rabies isolate. Am J Vet Res 1998;59:1629–32.
[32] Li X, Fox JG, Padrid PA. Neoplastic diseases in ferrets: 574 cases (1968–1997). J Am Vet Med Assoc 1998;212:1402–6.
[33] Dillberger JE, Altman NH. Neoplasia in ferrets: eleven cases with a review. J Comp Pathol 1989;100:161–76.
[34] Hanley CS, Wilson GH, Frank P, et al. T cell lymphoma in the lumbar spine of a domestic ferret (Mustela putorius futo). Vet Rec 2004;329–32.
[35] Erdman SE, Brown SA, Kawasaki TA, et al. Clinical and pathological findings in ferrets with lymphoma: 60 cases (1982–1994). J Am Vet Med Assoc 1996;208:1285–9.
[36] Dunn DG, Harris RK, Meis JM, et al. A histomorphologic and immunohistochemical study of chordoma in twenty ferrets (Mustela putorius futo). Vet Pathol 1991;28:467–73.
[37] Roth L, Takata I. Cytological diagnosis of chordoma of the tail in a ferret. Vet Clin Pathol 1992;21:119–21.
[38] Allison N, Rakich P. Chordoma in two ferrets. J Comp Pathol 1988;98:371–4.
[39] Herron AJ, Brunnert SR, Ching SV, et al. Immonohistochemical and morphologic features of chordomas in ferrets (Mustela putorius futo). Vet Pathol 1990;27:284–6.
[40] Hendrick MJ, Goldschmidt MH. Chondrosarcoma in the tail of ferrets. Vet Pathol 1987;24: 272–3.
[41] Williams BH, Eighmy JJ, Berbert MH, et al. Cervical chordoma in two ferrets. Vet Pathol 1993;30:204–6.
[42] Munday JS, Brown CA, Richey LJ. Suspected metastatic coccygeal chordoma in a ferret (Mustela putorius futo). J Vet Diagn Invest 2004;16:454–8.
[43] Pye GW, Bennett RA, Roberts GD, et al. Thoracic veterbral chordoma in a domestic ferret (Mustela putorius futo). J Zoo Wildl Med 2000;31:107–11.
[44] Jensen WA, Myers RK, Liu C-H. Osteoma in a ferret. J Am Vet Med Assoc 1985;187: 1375–6.
[45] Ryland LM, Gogolewski R. What's your diagnosis? J Am Vet Med Assoc 1990;197:1065–6.
[46] De Voe RS, Pack L, Greenacre CB. Radiographic and CT imaging of a skull associated osteoma in a ferret. Vet Radiol Ultrasound 2002;43:346–8.
[47] Sleeman JM, Clyde VL, Brenneman KA. Granular cell tumor in the central nervous system of a ferret (Mustela putorius futo). Vet Rec 1996;138:65–6.

[48] Frederick MA. Intervertebral disc syndrome in a domestic ferret. Vet Med Small Anim Clin 1981;76:835.

[49] Lu D, Lamb CR, Patterson-Kane JC, et al. Treatment of a prolapsed lumbar intervertebral disc in a ferret. J Small Anim Pract 2004;45:501–3.

[50] Morera N, Valls X, Mascort J. Intervertebral disc prolapse in a ferret. Vet Clin North Am Exot Anim Pract 2006;9:667–71.

[51] Fox JG, Zeeman DH, Mortimer JD. Copper toxicosis in sibling ferrets. J Am Vet Med Assoc 1994;205:1154–6.

[52] Williams BH, Popek EJ, et al. Iniencephaly and other neural tube defects in a litter of ferrets. Vet Path 1994;31:260–2.

[53] Lewington JH. Parasitic diseases of ferrets. In: Lewington JH, editor. Ferret husbandry, medicine, and surgery. 1st edition. Woburn (MA): Butterworth Heinemann; 2000. p. 129–52.

[54] Fox JG. Parasitic diseases. In: Fox JG, editor. Biology and diseases of the ferret. 2nd edition. Baltimore (MD): Lippincott Williams and Wilkins; 1998. p. 375–91.

ELSEVIER
SAUNDERS

VETERINARY
CLINICS
Exotic Animal Practice

Vet Clin Exot Anim 10 (2007) 775–802

Avian Neuroanatomy Revisited: From Clinical Principles to Avian Cognition

Susan E. Orosz, PhD, DVM,
DABVP (Avian), DECAMS[a],*,
G.A. Bradshaw, PhD[b,c]

[a]Bird and Exotic Pet Wellness Center, 5166 Monroe Street,
Suite 305, Toledo, OH 43623, USA
[b]The Kerulos Centre for Animal Psychology and Trauma Recovery,
Environmental Science Graduate Program,
Oregon State University, Corvallis, OR 95331, USA
[c]Pacifica Graduate Institute, Carpinteria, CA 93013, USA

On the surface, and in real ways, birds and mammals are very different. Aside from eccentrics like the platypus, bills, beaks, eggs, and feathers are foreign to the mammalian world. Birds also have been regarded as lower than mammals, lagging in the progress of evolution, and lacking in the neuroanatomical machinery that enables complex behavior and cognition—hence the less than complimentary epithet of bird brain.

Today, however, huge strides in avian neuroscience and ethology have changed this view and brought a deeper appreciation for their abilities. Cortex neuroanatomy and cytoarchitecture indicate that the evolution of mammalian and avian neural substrates may have diverged, but mental evolution has been convergent [1]. New research on neuroanatomy, coupled with ethological evidence, has demonstrated that avian cognition is on par with that of mammals. For instance, attributes such as linguistic ability, spatial memory, social reasoning, personality, representation of self, tool manipulation, episodic memory, and vocal learning [2–9] observed in avian species are considered comparable to those in primates. Further, brain structures underlying these abilities and responsible for processing emotional and social information and their associated traits (eg, maternal behavior, communication and conspecific recognition, play, sexual behavior, fear,

Portions of this work appeared originally in Orosz SE, Principles of avian clinical neuroanatomy. Semin Avian Exotic Pet Med 1996;5(3):127–39; reprinted with permission.

* Corresponding author.
E-mail address: drsusanorosz@aol.com (S.E. Orosz).

aggression, and affect regulation) are all highly conserved evolutionarily across species (Table 1) [10]. Birds are not just a step ahead of reptiles, nor are they emotionally immature, but closer to being feathered apes [11].

Concurrent with these avian discoveries, the entire field of neurosciences has been undergoing its own evolution. Determinants of behavior are seen as products of nature (genes) and nurture (environment). Formerly regarded as primitive reflexes, emotions have gained greater status in the broader scheme of mental processing and now are understood to interact seamlessly with cognition in vital survival functions including stress regulation, perception, social processing, and complex decision making [12]. There is now an entire subfield, affective neuroscience, devoted to the study of the neural substrates underlying emotion and feelings [10].

What emerges is a picture of the brain as an integrated mosaic of distributed, interacting cognitive and affective processes that are informed through relational transactions in the environment. The brain is cognitive, emotional, and social, whose core mechanisms and structures are describable by common, cross-taxa models of brain and behavior [13–16]. All of these insights are changing how avian behavior is envisioned, and subsequently how a bird is approached clinically. This article begins with a brief review of: (1) new models of the brain and its evolution and (2) relationships between sociality, brain development, and stress affects, and how they inform the understanding of avian cognition, behavior, and health.

New models of the avian brain and its evolution

In the long-held view of neuroanatomy, there was an evolutionary hierarchy that suggested lower vertebrates (fish, reptiles, and birds) had poor cognitive abilities and operated basically by reflexes. The unified theory of brain evolution embraced by Edinger and others [1] implied a linear evolution of the brain and concomitant evolution of higher level thinking as one progressed up the evolutionary ladder from fish to people (ie, *scala naturae*).

Table 1
Comparable anatomical structures for mammalian and avian brains

Mammalian	Avian
Prefrontal neocortex	Nidopallium
Ophthalmic division (V1), primary visual cortex, and somatosensory cortex	Wulst (entopallium)
Associative cortex	Mesopallium
Primary auditory cortex	Field L
Amygdala	Amygdaloid complex
Thalamus	Thalamus
Cerebellum	Cerebellum
Hypothalamic-pituitary-adrenal axis (HPA)	HPA
Hippocampus	Hippocampus

This way of thinking suggested that parts of the brain were older, and as evolution progressed, there would be newer and more complex components added. This linear view resulted in subdivisions of the brain from older, less complex regions such as the paleostriatum and archistriatum, to the newer portions termed the neostriatum, suggesting a neocortex for the brain of mammals.

A misinterpretation of Greek terms, however, led to erroneous nomenclature. Although paleo means ancient or primitive it does not imply the oldest. Archi in Greek means oldest, the first, or the most primitive, but it was relegated to the position after paleo in the terms used for classification. The ability to interpret and think in a social context was thought to reside only in the neocortex, suggesting that birds had, at best, limited ability to have those higher-level faculties.

The avian brain and brain stem were considered to have evolved from the reptilian brain. The caudal portion of the brain, the brain stem (medulla, pons, and midbrain or mesencephalon), evolved similarly in both birds and in mammals (Fig. 1). The rostral portion or prosencephalon (telencephalon and diencephalon), however, evolved differently in birds compared with mammals. The area associated with the cortex was thought to evolve from a reptilian archistratum or archaic striatum above the paleostriatum. This structure was proposed as the precursor of the human caudate and putamen, which represent subcortical nuclei associated with the quality of movement. The paleostriatum of reptiles was to have an older part or primitivum and a newer portion, the augmentatum. Both of these subdivisions were considered homologous to the globus pallidus of people, part of the subcortical nuclei associated with smooth execution of willful movement. Birds were thought to have uniquely evolved a newer component to the basal ganglia, the hyperstriatum or hypertrophied striatum [1].

But the animals below the mammals were not supposed to have developed a cortex with its amazing ability to think beyond reflexes. Reptiles had an archicortex that was mainly olfactory in function and considered primitive at best. Birds also were considered in the same category. It was only the mammals that were to evolve the greatest achievement, a neocortex of six layers from the two- to three-layered plan of the primitive subcortical archi and paleocortex of these lower animals [1].

Recent advances in the understanding of brain evolution, however, have radically changed the way of thinking neuroanatomically. Enzyme studies of neuroreceptors, anatomic profiles of gene products, and studies on avian cognition and brain function have lead to new terminology from the Avian Brain Nomenclature Consortium [1]. This terminology reflects the current understanding of vertebrate brain organization, homologies, evolution, and function. This new terminology scheme facilitates a greater understanding of brain function in birds and no longer inhibits study design that gets to the core of avian cognition, as well as a better understanding of emotional tone [1].

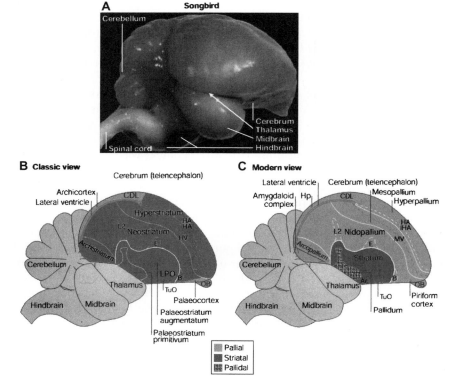

Fig. 1. Side view of a zebra finch, demonstrating the physical external brain (*A*), the classic view of its structure (*B*), and the modern consensus view from the Avian Brian Nomenclature Forum. (*From* Jarvis ED, Gunturkun O, Bruce L, et al. Perspectives. Avian brains and a new understanding of vertebrate brain evolution. The Avian Brain Nomenclature Consortium. Nat Rev Neurosci 2005;6:151–9; with permission.)

One of the current authors (SEO) suggested previously that the functional neuroanatomical homologies do not suggest that birds are limited only to an instinctual level of function [17]. She suggested that although the brains of birds appear different anatomically from people, functions performed in the brain remained similar. The cerebral cortex of a bird or reptile brain is lissencephalic, meaning that it is smooth-surfaced and not punctuated by gyri and sulci, a feature of the neocortex of mammals (Fig. 2). The cortical cells of mammals that process information developed on the surface, whereas the homologous cells were retained deep within the cortex in birds and reptiles in the subcortical nuclei. This did not necessarily mean that bird brains were or are stupid! They just process the information in a different location and manner (ie, using three-layered subcortical nuclei, not a six-layered cortex).

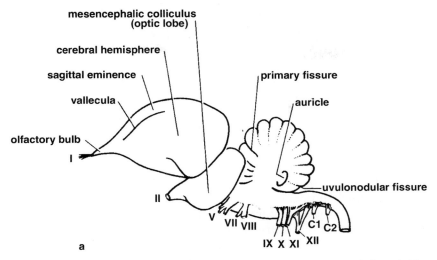

Fig. 2. Lateral view of the brain of a domestic chicken, with cranial nerves indicated. (*From* King AS, McClelland J. Birds: their structure and function. 2nd edition. Bath (United Kingdom): Bailliere Tindall; 1984. p. 237–314.)

Sociality, brain development, and stress

The stress response

In its most general definition, stress results from a differential between ourselves and what is around us. Every species, and individual, has a particular evolutionary, ecological, and experientially shaped envelope of tolerance within which they live more or less comfortably. Each has specific coping strategies that adjust behavior, physiology, and neurobiology to accommodate stressor effects [18].

Two major systems mediate the stress response: the hypothalamic-pituitary-adrenocortical (HPA) system or axis, which stimulates the adrenal cortex to release glucocorticoids (eg, cortisol, corticosterone) into the blood, and the sympathetic adrenomedullary system, which influences the stress response through parallel pathways [19]. Through the process of allostasis (ie, maintenance of stability through change), the brain uses its extensive neuronal plasticity to successfully adapt to stressful circumstances and maintain homeostasis [20]. When stress becomes repeated or prolonged (ie, allostatic overload), the individual's adaptive threshold is exceeded, and adaptive capacity fails through an inability to accommodate. The result is potentially serious physical and/or psychological trauma.

Traumatic stress generally is distinguished from other stress in that it is defined as a physically or emotionally inflicted injury perceived by an individual or a group to threaten existence [21]. Chronic stress and psychobiological trauma manifest both intraorganismically (eg, increased vulnerability to disease and predisposition to injury) and interorganismically (eg, asocial and atypical affiliative behaviors) through triggering hyperarousal in the limbic and autonomic nervous systems. Such responses are most likely to occur when stressors are of a social nature. Social factors are powerful modulators of the stress response and can affect significant changes in neuroendocrinal system and behavior [22].

Neuroethology of social attachment and its disruption

Altricial vertebrates, including psittacine birds, are immersed in a social environment. Social attachment transactions occur throughout life with parents, nest mates, mates, and other flock members. These bonds provide primary external sources of sensory input and regulation of all essential developmental processes that interact with genetics and the greater environmental surround [23]. Diverse communication modalities (touch, smell, taste, sound, sight) form the sensory matrix in which the chick or infant is embedded and with which the chick's own autonomic nervous system (ANS) interacts [24].

Social development coincides with periods of rapid brain growth and shaping of affective and self-regulatory systems that guide the developing individual's stress responses through neuro–ethological patterning and tissue-specific effects on gene expression. Early experiences and context influence the HPA axis, hippocampus, and other parts of the brain [24–29].

Extensive, long-term studies have shown that without knowledge of ontogenetic social context, vocal and behavioral outcomes cannot be predicted [30]. How an individual initially develops affects viability and adaptation success over the entire life span [31,32]. Differences in neurochemical pathways are related to observable variations in behavior, sociality, and life histories (eg, prairie and montane voles [33,34].) One therefore can understand species-specific behavior (and dysfunctions) as reflective of underlying species-tailored neuroendocrinal patterns (eg, facial recognition and song processing in mammals and oscines, respectively [7]). For example, the need for young of altricial species to be able to process complex social (eg, communication) and ecological (eg, foraging) information is expressed in the significant postnatal differentiation of the brain and neural pathways and stress sensitivity [35]. The fact that many of behavioral disorders in captive birds tend to present in one taxa preferentially over another (eg, self-mutilation in cockatoos) is consistent with the link between neuroendocrinal pathways and species-species patterns of sociality [34].

When social stress occurs, and normative processes of attachment are disrupted, prolonged or acute HPA axis activation and associated elevated endogenous corticosteroids occur. Severe stress can impair gene expression involved in neurogenesis and synaptogenesis and compromise maturing brain circuits involved in mnemonic, cognitive and affective regulatory functions [36]. Traumatic disruption from a single threatening event alone can create lifelong changes in social learning abilities and neural organization (eg, the genesis of stereotypies and concomitant compromise to basal ganglia [37,38]).

Direct (eg, death of mother, impaired rearing) or indirect (eg, transmitted maternal stress) compromise may induce sustained effects on brain plasticity and create a structural vulnerability for psychopathogenesis, early death, or behavioral dysfunction [39]. Deviations from normative social interactions therefore translate to altered patterns in core survival functions that govern coping behavior and stress regulation abilities.

In mammals, stress effects are not limited to direct experience but can transmit across generations: relational stress during gestational and postnatal periods can pass to offspring [27]. Resulting impairment of socio–affective circuits, especially in higher cortical regions, underlie many abnormal and inappropriate emotional responses. These can express at later stages of life biochemically as elevated levels of arousal regulating catecholamines, corticotropin-releasing factor, and corticosteroids and expressed behaviorally in one or more ways:

A persistent fearful temperament
Diminished capacity to modulate memory, fear, and social judgment
A predisposition to aggression dysregulation and violence
Post-traumatic stress disorder (PTSD) [32]

These etiologies may relate to the sudden appearance of phobic behavior prevalent in many hand-reared parrots: feather-picking, mate trauma, and sudden, seemingly unprovoked aggression and screaming [31,40–42].

Clinical implications

A consideration of stress physiology and developmental neurobiology raises several important points in clinical assessment. First, these concepts imply that, in principle, all companion bird psychophysiological envelopes potentially are exceeded on a regular basis. Most, if not all, wild and domestic captive companion avian species that enter the clinic live in conditions significantly different from those to which they are evolutionarily and ecologically adapted. Most captive conditions deviate hugely from the foraging, food consumed, sociality, and habitat of wild free-ranging species. This implies that birds in captivity are vulnerable to excessive levels and types of stress relative to their natural capacities, thereby potentially leading to a perennial susceptibility to disease. Furthermore, captivity by definition disallows what traumatologists consider to be a key factor in maintaining psychophysiological integrity: agency or free will [21,43].

Most companion birds, particularly those that are long-lived, experience not one but typically a series of traumatic disruptions in their lifetime: premature weaning, compromised rearing (eg, hand-rearing), social disruption through premature weaning, separation from conspecific or human companions (eg, relinquishment to new home), and impoverished socio–eco-logical conditions and isolation (eg, barren cage living with little enrichment or social interactions). Captivity needs to be understood as an ongoing stressor that can threaten the well-being of companion birds.

Behavioral and physical presentations may relate directly or indirectly to a history of neurophysiological compromise (eg, feather-damaging behavior, human–bird bond problems). For this reason, it may not always be possible to eradicate, or necessarily readily diagnose complications from the effects of early or chronic trauma. Repeated, prolonged stress can result in complex PTSD: a condition whose symptoms are diffuse, difficult to diagnosis, and tenacious. Symptoms include personality disturbances such as identity confusion, self-injurious behavior, depression, social and physical incompetence, and attachment disorders (Table 2) [43]. Symptoms commonly observed in abused or neglected companion parrots (eg, feather-damaging behavior, eating disorders, hyperaggression, agitated screaming, stereotypy, mate trauma, and unresponsiveness) are consistent with symptoms of complex PSTD and other trauma-induced behaviors.

Treatment

What can be done to reduce stress in a captive environment and even address past trauma? In the realm of human recovery, where most of the theory and practice have been detailed, diverse methods are employed. There is a basic set of goals, however, upon which nearly all health professionals agree: to create conditions that support overall health and well-being, a sense of relaxation and security, social bonding, agency, competence, self-esteem, and the prevention of threat and domination (Box 1) [43].

Table 2
Complex post-traumatic stress disorder symptoms and characteristics for people

Symptom	Characteristics for people
Attachment	Problems with boundaries
	Distrust and suspiciousness
	Asociality
Biology	Sensorimotor developmental problems
	Increased medical problems across a wide span
Affect regulation	Difficulty with emotional self-regulation
Dissociation	Depersonalization and derealization
Behavioral control	Aggression against others
	Pathological self-injurious behaviors
	Sleep disturbances
	Eating disorders
Cognition	Anhedonia
	Lack of sustained curiosity
	Learning difficulties
	Acoustic and visual perceptual problems

Data from Herman J. Trauma and recovery. New York: Basic Books; 1997.

Box 1. Trauma restoration and treatment goals for people

Agency, self-efficacy, mastery, perceived control
Self-esteem, hope, and optimism
Relaxation, competence, and assertiveness
Ability to tell your story (developing a coherent narrative),
    participatory listening
Inter- or intraspecific bonding
Health and well-being
Avoidance of isolation and marginalization
No threats or domination (mutual facilitation)
Healthy, safe living environment
Support personal change in mood, diet, behavior, and social
    alliance changes

Many practices currently recommended for companion birds are consistent with those employed for human trauma survivors [43,44]. For example, creating a living environment that matches the bird's natural ecology significantly decreases environmental stress. Situations and foods that resemble the nutrition, shape, and texture of their habitat and habits emulate the conditions to which they are evolutionarily, ecologically, and experientially adapted. Since captivity generally reduces the amount of exercise and movement characteristic of free-ranging conditions, achieving good health for the companion bird also includes allowing the bird to move, fly, and interact much as they do in the wild. Being able to be a bird in all the diverse ways builds physical competence and therefore psychological competence. Such a natural environment conforms to their envelope of tolerance and relative comfort.

Close attention needs to be paid to species' and individual differences. African gray parrots naturally bathe while foraging along stream banks, but Amazon parrots on the other hand bathe as a consequence of often-occurring rain showers. Therefore providing shallow bathing pools with river rocks for foraging helps African gray parrots mimic their natural behaviors, while showering Amazons daily overhead mimics their natural behavior.

Healthful living conditions include the social dimension. The psittacine world is a social world. Strong, consistent, lifelong relationships not only nurture emotional and physical well-being, but also help buffer life events and other stressful episodes that can tax an individual significantly (eg, death of mate).

In most cases, the most important relationship is the primary human caregiver. Whether or not the bird is a social obligate (eg, parrots), the human caregiver is crucial. The caregiver is the source of food, home, and security—or not. This relational dependency, therefore, confers great importance. The quality of this relationship reflects how a bird feels about his/her environment. Is home secure or dangerous and threatening? As neuroscience shows, chronic uncertainty translates to chronic stress and increases the potential for retraumatization. Feeding at similar times of the day and having a regular schedule may help to reduce uncertainty and stress. Similar to the discussion on biophysical conditions, there are significant species and individual differences.

Certain species appear to handle stress better. For example, bird species such as budgerigars and cockatiels, which have been bred in captivity for long periods of time, generally appear to handle life with people better. On the other hand, African gray parrots and the most cockatoo species do not appear as adaptable as evidenced by their common presentations of feather damaging behaviors.

This article discussed earlier that captivity by definition disallows agency (free will). Much can be accomplished within these bounds, however, by encouraging natural behavior and the ability to make decisions and choices. Restoring agency means supporting a bird so that it can be a bird when, how, and where it wants. Simply being able to choose its own food, to eat when it wants, to visit with friends when it wishes, always having the choice to engage or not engage in an activity, and to be able to explore its habitat at will is psychologically and physically restorative. This freedom encourages confidence and a sense of mastery and control.

Obviously, achieving these goals can create a significant demand on the human caregiver: branch chewing in the wild does not find much support when in captivity the object of an Amazon's beak is an elegant chair. Another natural behavior is the Amazon that screams shortly after sunup and before sundown to call the flock. That normal behavior often is misinterpreted by owners. Once again, principles of psychobiology bring attention to a critical point: behavior and health are contingent on both the state of mind (psyche) and state of the body (biology). It is not only the physical and ecological aspects of a bird's world that affect well-being (eg, branches for climbing and bark stripping and natural play with objects containing food can address psychophysiological needs). Well-being also is affected by the quality that the caregiver brings to the environment. This is a subtle and critical point. It is in and through relationships that the trauma of captivity occurs (eg, capture, abandonment, abusive neglect), and therefore it is through the establishment of a secure, trusting, and liberating relationship that progress of recovery can be made. Threat and domination characterize and enable traumatization, and it is their absence that opens the opportunity for healing. The opposite of domination and threat is mutuality and trust: qualities that neuroscience identifies as essential for the caretaker to cultivate for supporting agency, competence, and well-being.

There is one goal considered pivotal in human recovery that the authors have not addressed here: the opportunity of someone who has been silenced and denied an existence other than that dictated by his or her captor, to speak of his or her experience [21,43]. The idea of a parrot telling its story may sound guilty of egregious anthropomorphism, but given what is known of neurobiological and behavioral similarities, how might one envision a translation across species? Trauma psychologists expand symptom beyond pathology and reframe behavioral disorders as communications of suffering and distress [43]. Extrapolating to companion birds, misbehavior is not merely a problem to get rid of, but contains valuable information of the bird's past experience and a psychophysiological communication that literally embodies their story: "the body keeps the score" [21].

In short, much can be done to help ameliorate conditions and experience of stress. Nonetheless, although many stress-induced dysfunctions may be addressed with good supportive, nurturing care, a long-term predilection for psychological and physiological compromise may endure. This is important to communicate to the human guardian who needs to know that while cognitive–behavioral approaches and environmental manipulations will reduce undesirable behaviors, there is a potential for them to resurface under stress.

As mentioned earlier, diagnosis of trauma- and stress-induced disorders can be diffuse and appear systemic rather than reveal as a specific lesion. A general physical and behavioral examination included with the bird's biography can provide substantive information on sequelae and events, however. The authors now review clinically relevant anatomy of the avian central nervous system that is necessary to accurately perform the neurological examination, better interpret findings, and localize lesions.

The central nervous system

To localize a lesion in the central nervous system, the clinician must understand at least several of the long ascending and descending tracts and the location of the cranial nerve nuclei in the brain and brain stem. This discussion will focus on the neuroanatomic principles of birds important to avian veterinarians for handling neurological problems.

The most important anatomical information concerning the brain stem for the avian clinician is the location and function of the cranial nerve nuclei. This understanding, combined with the knowledge of the major ascending or sensory and descending or motor tracts, will help the avian veterinarian determine if the lesion that he or she observes can be localized. The following description of the cranial nerve nuclei will orient the avian veterinarian to the components of the brainstem to localize lesions to a specific portion of the CNS, and will help those reading advanced radiological images.

Spinal cord

The spinal cord of birds is basically the same length as its vertebral column [30]. Therefore, the spinal cord segment is at the same level as its vertebral column segment. Spinal nerves pass laterally through the vertebral foramina rather than caudally. This anatomic finding makes it easier to localize a lesion in birds than in mammals. Because the spinal cord is as long as the neural canal, birds do not have a cauda equina. Therefore, myelograms are more difficult to perform.

There are two potential enlargements of the spinal cord grossly. Most birds have a cervical and a lumbosacral enlargement. Birds that fly have a cervical enlargement that is more pronounced than their lumbosacral enlargement. On the other hand, it is the authors' observation that ratites, and presumably birds that have fine motor control of their legs and toes, have a more pronounced lumbosacral enlargement.

In addition, birds have a unique structure in their lumbosacral cord [30,45,46]. In this region, the dorsal columns are separated laterally, and the space created contains the glycogen body. This body consists of a collection of periependymal glycogen cells with nests of argentafin cells. In addition, there are numerous nerve terminals that are basically of two anatomic types. One type of terminals appears to be sensory, and the nerve fibers are related to both the periependymal glycogen cells and the adjacent capillaries. These nerve fibers may a play role in regulating vascular reflexes. The second type of nerve terminals forms a thick collection that ends on blood capillaries within the middle of the glycogen body. These fibers are believed to have a neurosecretory role [46].

There are other anatomic features of the spinal cord that are unique to birds. The meninges consist of pia, arachnoid, and dura mater as in mammals [30]. Birds differ, however, in that the dura is separated from the periosteal lining, forming an epidural space in the cervical and thoracic regions. This space is filled with a gelatinous tissue that is believed to act as a shock absorber. Its gelatinous nature would be particularly important in birds, owing to the enhanced flexibility of their necks compared with mammals [30]. Birds require this mobility to compensate for their reduced ability to use their thoracic limbs for manipulation. Instead, they use their bills for such activities as grooming and nest building.

In addition, birds have in their spinal canals long and short suspensory ligaments in the region of the brachial plexus. These ligaments pass from the vertebral bodies to the nerve roots. They function to transmit tension from the spinal cord and nerve roots to the vertebral column during manipulation of the wings to absorb tensile forces [47]. Another unique feature of birds is that the internal vertebral venous plexus runs the entire length of the vertebral column [30]. This venous plexus is connected to the venous drainage of the kidney and may transmit infectious agents or tumor cells to other parts of the body.

The spinal cord of birds is divided into three white matter columns on each side that surround the central gray matter. These three columns of white matter tracts are divided into the dorsal column, the lateral column, and the ventral column. The dorsal column lies between the dorsal median septum and the rootlets of the dorsal horn [30,45]. The dorsal column is relatively small in birds compared with mammals, particularly primates. The lateral column is sandwiched between the dorsal and ventral horn with their emerging rootlets. The ventral column lies between the ventral median fissure and the ventral rootlets of the ventral horn. The ventral and lateral columns are relatively larger than the dorsal column in birds.

The gray matter of the spinal cord has the traditional butterfly-shaped appearance with the centrally located spinal canal. The ventral horn is larger than the dorsal horn, particularly in the cervical and lumbosacral enlargements, and accounts for the bulge observed grossly. In addition, birds have marginal nuclei that surround the outer margins of the butterfly of gray matter. They form a continuous column of gray matter and consist of multipolar neurons like those of the ventral horn cells. Although they may be ventral horn cells that have migrated laterally, they more likely appear to be ventral commissural neurons that project information from one side of the cord to the other [30]. Additionally, they may represent multisynaptic neurons that transmit nonlocalizing pain fibers up and down the column [48]. The gray matter of pigeons has been regionalized into seven areas that appear to be similar to the Rexed lamina of cats [30,48,49]. This anatomic homology adds further understanding of the nervous system functionally.

The long ascending pathways

The dorsal column (fasiculus gracilis and cuneatus of mammals)
The dorsal column [30,45,48,49] consists of a collection of white matter fibers that originate from afferent neurons whose cell bodies are in the dorsal root ganglion. Although the exact modalities are unknown in birds, it is assumed that they contain information from the body wall related to touch, pressure, and kinesthesia or proprioception of the joints. As in mammals, these modalities of discriminative touch, pressure, and kinesthesia are believed to be arranged somatotopically in the dorsal column [48,49]. This means that the information from the caudal region is carried more medially in the column, whereas the more proximal areas are more lateral. This column in birds is uniform in width [30,45], suggesting that many of the axons are short or move to another location in the cord. These fibers end in the nucleus gracilis or cuneatus in the medulla. Axons from these two nuclei ascend laterally as the medial lemniscus in the brain stem to end predominantly in the thalamus [30,45]. From here, the thalamic projections most likely ascend to the hyperstriatum (new classification: mesopallium) and neostriatum (new classification: nidopallium) of the telencephalon, where the bird can perceive touch and pressure and discriminate its location on the body wall [17].

Dorsolateral ascending bundle (dorsal spinocerebellar tract of mammals)
Although this bundle [30,34,48,49] receives some fibers from the ventral ascending bundle, for simplicity's sake, the dorsolateral bundle can be

considered homologous to the dorsal spinocerebellar tract [30,48,49]. The nerve fibers that make up this tract are homologous to Clarke's column, which sends information from muscle receptors in mammals to the cerebellum from the same side of the body or ipsilaterally. In birds, unconscious proprioception is confined to the wing [17,30,45].

Ventrolateral ascending bundle (ventral spinocerebellar tract of mammals)

This bundle of fibers [30,45,48,49] is activated by muscle afferents of the hind limb. They enter the cord where they decussate to ascend as the ventrolateral ascending bundle. These fibers are believed to cross again as in mammals in the rostral cerebellar peduncle. Like the dorsolateral ascending bundle, the information concerning unconscious proprioception of the body is believed to be organized ipsilaterally with respect to the cerebellar hemispheres. The information that is transmitted to the cerebellum then is used to formulate a plan for motor activity of the body [17].

Dorsolateral fasiculus (tract of Lissauer or spinothalamic)

There is a small collection of fibers that caps the tip of the dorsal horn. These fibers end on the nucleus at this tip of the horn, the nucleus substantia gelatinosa. Its homology in mammals is the tract of Lissauer or the lateral spinothalamic tract [30,45,48,49]. Fibers concerned with pain, temperature, and light touch in mammals synapse in the substantia gelatinosa, decussate, and then ascend as the spinothalamic tract in the lateral column of the spinal cord and brainstem to the thalamus. In pigeons, this tract has similar neuroanatomic pathways but appears to transmit tactile information only [47].

Spinoreticular tract

The spinoreticular tract ascends bilaterally in the reticular formation to the medulla, pons, and mesecephalon [30]. It is believed to be somatosensory for the delivery of information concerned with pain.

Propriospinal system (fasiculus proprius of mammals)

This propriospinal system [45–47] consists of short fibers that are polysynaptic and ascend up the spinal cord to the reticular formation. This system cannot discriminate the precise location of noxious stimuli; instead, it makes one aware of a vague sense of pain that is nonlocalizable.

From these descriptions and their considered homologs, one can see that the nervous system of birds is complex and has the ability to perceive noxious stimuli and hence pain, an important consideration in veterinary medicine.

The long descending pathway

The long descending pathways of birds are not as well known as those of the ascending ones. It is believed that many of the tracts are long

spinal–spinal pathways. The intricate and precise movements of birds, however, would suggest that there are important tracts that influence alpha motoneurons to perform these activities.

Lateral reticulospinal tract (lateral reticulospinal tract of mammals)

This tract [30,48,49] appears to be homologous to the lateral tract of mammals. It originates in the reticular formation of the brain stem and ends at the nucleus intermedius. The nucleus intermedius of mammals represents the preganglionic cell bodies of the autonomic motor system. It is believed that this tract in birds also is concerned with visceral motor function [17].

Rubrospinal tract (rubrospinal tract of mammals)

This tract [30,45,48,49] is the other motor tract in the lateral column. It takes origin in the red nucleus of the mesencephalon and decussates near its origin before continuing through the brain stem. This tract ends near the alpha motoneurons in the ventral horn of the gray matter. The red nucleus is believed to be organized somatotopically. These fibers enhance flexor tone of skeletal muscles [17].

Cerebrospinal tract (pyramidal tract of mammals)

Studies suggest that there is a long tract that originates in the archistriatum or archopallium in the forebrain. This tract [30,48,49] is believed to decussate in the pyramids of the ventral medulla to descend in both the ventral and dorsal columns. As in ungulates, it is believed to be limited to providing upper motor neuron input to the alpha motoneurons in the ventral horn of the cervical region only [17].

Vestibulospinal tract (vestibulospinal tract of mammals)

The vestibulospinal tract [30,48,49] can be divided into two: a medial tract that is larger than a lateral one. The medial tract is believed to be homologous to the ventral vestibulospinal tract. The lateral one represents the vestibulospinal tract of mammals. These two tracts run the length of the spinal cord in the ventral column. Both are believed to stimulate extensor tone of skeletal muscles. They arise, in part, from the medial longitudinal fasiculus, a white matter tract predominantly of the brain stem that coordinates eye movement. Flight and the ability to move freely in three-dimensional space would require the bird to be able to coordinate eye and body movements quickly [17].

Reticulospinal tract (medial reticulospinal tract of mammals)

The reticulospinal tract [30,48,49] arises from pontine reticular nuclei and descends in the ipsilateral spinal cord. Its function in birds is unknown, but it is believed to be involved in altering somatic and visceral motor tone.

Tectospinal tract (tectospinal tract of mammals)

As the name implies, the tract [30,48,49] originates in the optic tectum and descends to at least the cervical region of the spinal cord. This tract is involved in the coordination of reflex movements between the eyes and the upper body, particularly the neck.

Olfactory nerve (cranial nerve I)

The olfactory nerve [30,50] is made up of afferent fibers whose cell bodies are found predominantly within the epithelium of the caudal nasal conchae (Fig. 3). These scrolls of cartilage with an overlying epithelium project from the lateral walls of the nasal cavity. The degree of scrolling varies, with those birds that have greater olfactory perception having more highly developed conchae with extensive folding. The bipolar ciliated neuronal cells that make up the olfactory nerve are supported by basal and sustentacular cells.

This olfactory epithelium is found not only in the caudal nasal conchae but also may be found in the dorsal and lateral walls of the nasal cavity, as well as in the nasal septum. The afferent unmyelinated fibers of cranial

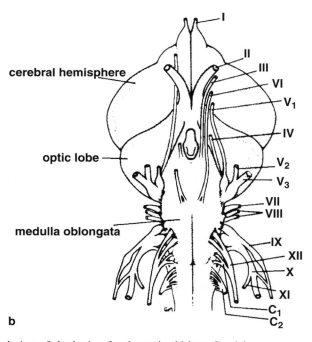

Fig. 3. Ventral view of the brain of a domestic chicken. Cranial nerves are represented by roman numerals. C_1 and C_2 are the first and second cervical spinal nerves. (*From* King AS, McClelland J. Birds: their structure and function. 2nd edition. Bath (United Kingdom): Bailliere Tindall; 1984. p. 237–314.)

nerve (CN) I enter the skull through a foramen (the olfactory foramen) as opposed to the cribriform plate of mammals. They synapse at the olfactory bulb before entering the rostral cortex, usually by way of two centers.

It appears that olfaction in birds is similar to mammals as even passerines, an order of birds with the least olfactory capabilities, have behavioral responses to odors. Olfaction is used in numerous bird species to locate food. The black-footed albatross can smell bacon at a range of 20 miles from its source on the open ocean [51].

Other birds known to locate food using olfaction include vultures, ravens, crows, hummingbirds, and kiwis. Olfaction is used for navigational cueing in pigeons, as a means to locate nesting burrows in procellariiformes, and for reproductive behaviors in various species. Male ducks require olfaction for reproductive displays [52], and the odors of fruit in doves are important for normal care of the squabs [53]. There also is evidence of olfaction serving in the selection of the nesting materials that act to fumigate the nest for ectoparasites and various pathogens [54–57].

Complete sectioning of the olfactory nerve has been used experimentally for determining function, but the information can be used as a clinical gauge. Olfactory nerves were found to grow back after complete section, and the birds regained full physiologic capacity [58]. The nerves may be smaller and may have neuromas with scar tissue, but they have been able to detect odors to the same level as controls [58,59].

Optic nerve (cranial nerve II)

Birds are exquisitely visual animals. The cross-sectional diameter of the optic nerve is larger than the cross-sectional diameter of the cervical spinal cord. The optic nerve is developed best in falconiformes and least in nocturnal species. The afferent fibers from the ganglion cells of the retina become myelinated as they penetrate the sclera of the eye. The fibers course caudally through the optic foramen, and then almost all of them decussate at the optic chiasm before traveling to several locations.

Many of the fibers travel to areas that are involved with interpretation of the optic stimulus. Other fibers travel to the tectum, which is the superior colliculus in mammals. In birds, this tectum is so large that it has been termed the optic lobe. This large collection of nerve fibers and cells lies dorsal to the midbrain just rostral to the cerebellum.

The system associated with the optic lobe represents the centrifugal pathway and contains two cell groups: the isthmo–optic nucleus (ION) and the ectopic isthmo–optic neurons (EION). In seed and fruit eaters, the ION appears large, well differentiated, and laminated, and it is arranged somatotopically [60]. In raptors, these cell bodies are small, suggesting this system is associated with pecking and visual food selection of static stimuli. Other studies, however, demonstrated profound deficits in the detection of moving stimuli and grain on a checkerboard pattern when the cells of this area were lesioned. These data suggest that, like in mammals, this centrifugal system plays an important role in detecting moving objects and enhancing contrast under dim lighting conditions [61].

The tectofugal system consists of axons from the optic nerve that decussate and travel to the optic tectum but then project bilaterally to the thalamic nucleus rotundus before traveling to the ipsilateral ectostriatum. From here, there are multiple synapses as information travels to forebrain structures for interpretation of the visual field. Lesions of the tectum produce deficits in pattern and color discrimination.

Although clinically this may be hard to discern, careful examination of a bird considered to be blind must include a greater understanding of what constitutes blindness. Is the bird totally blind, or unable to perceive moving or static objects, or not able to perceive color? This gets into the discrimination of cortical versus peripheral blindness. Blindness is difficult to assess clinically. One test is the eye blink, where an object is flashed toward the bird. The sensory component to this test is the optic nerve, while the motor component for the blink is from cranial nerve V, not VII as in mammals. Birds, particularly raptors, can be very stoic and may not blink. The consensual and direct light response in mammals has dilation and pupillary constriction associated with shining a light into the eye. The sensory component is the optic nerve or cranial nerve II. The motor response for the constriction of the pupil is from cranial nerve III or the oculomotor nerve to the smooth muscle to the ciliary body of the pupil. Unfortunately in birds, the oculomotor nerve to the ciliary body controls skeletal muscle, not smooth muscle, so that it can override the system willfully and not constrict the pupil (Fig. 4).

This makes clinical diagnosis of blindness more difficult in birds compared with mammals. Taking birds into a dimly lit room should cause pupillary dilation. Turning the lights on after dilation can result in the bird suddenly constricting the pupils where both should be of equal size. This would require the anatomic pathway as described previously with the sensory component from CN II and the motor component from CN III. Taking the bird into a room with normal lighting but with unfamiliar objects scattered in its path will help to discern if the bird is blind. This also will determine if the avian patient can see objects at rest. When using moving objects to test for normal function of CN II and the optic tectum, most are of sufficient density to cause air movements that birds can easily perceive the turbulence created using general somatic afferents. Gently dropping cotton balls or large but lightweight objects helps to determine if the bird can see.

Oculomotor nerve (cranial nerve III)

CN III [30,48,50,62] represents the fibers that arise from the four parts of the oculomotor nucleus. This nucleus resides near the cerebral aqueduct of the ventricular system in the proximal midbrain. It is medial to the long ascending and descending white matter tracts. The oculomotor nerve enters the

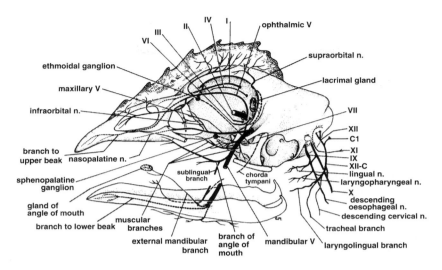

Fig. 4. Cranial nerves of the domestic chicken. The midregion of the left jugal arch has been removed. The sensory component of the eye is the optic nerve, or cranial nerve (CN) II, while the motor response to constrict the pupil is from the oculomotor nerve, or CN III. The trochlear nerve, CN IV, emerges from the trochlear foramen to innervate the dorsal oblique muscle of the eye, which moves the eye down and out. *Abbreviations:* C1, first cervical spinal nerve; n, nerve; Roman numerals, cranial nerves. (*From* King AS, McClelland J. Birds: their structure and function. 2nd edition. Bath (United Kingdom): Bailliere Tindall; 1984. p. 237–314.)

orbit through the oculomotor foramen. Three of its four components supply the extrinsic muscles of the eye. The fourth component provides the parasympathetic supply to the eye as the mammalian homolog, the Edinger-Westphal nucleus. This parasympathetic component innervates the intrinsic muscles of the eye (smooth muscle component), which also have voluntary control of pupillary constriction and dilation of the skeletal muscle to the ciliary body and the iris. The oculomotor nerve divides into a dorsal branch that innervates the dorsal rectus to the globe and the levator palpebrae superioris muscle, which elevates the upper lid. This muscle contains both skeletal and smooth muscle fibers. The oculomotor nerve has a ventral branch that supplies the ventral and medial rectus muscles, the ventral oblique muscles, and the ciliary ganglion. This ganglion represents the postganglionic parasympathetic cell bodies of CN III to smooth muscles of the eye. As described under CN II, constriction of the pupil is under the control of CN III. Dilation in birds often represents a disruption of this nerve to the eye or dysfunction of CN II. In mammals, dilation also can result from increased sympathetic tone.

Trochlear nerve (cranial nerve IV)

The nucleus of CN IV [30,48–50,62] is found just caudal to the oculomotor nucleus of CN III. Its nerve fibers emerge dorsally from the midbrain, the only cranial nerve to do so. The axons of this nerve decussate before traveling through the trochlear foramen to innervate the dorsal oblique muscle, an extrinsic eye muscle. Therefore, the muscle on the right side is controlled by the left nucleus in the midbrain, and vice versa for the other side (see Fig. 4). The dorsal oblique muscle moves the eye down and out in direction. Eye movement is restricted compared with mammals, however, so it is difficult to detect a lesion of this nerve or nucleus.

Trigeminal nerve (cranial nerve V)

There are multiple nuclei in the brainstem associated with cranial nerve V [30,48–50,62,63] or the trigeminal nerve (see Fig. 4), depending on function. There is a large nucleus that extends through the pons and is somatotopically arranged for receiving general somatic afferent information from the head. CN V enters the brainstem just caudal to the optic lobe, but ventrally. It is the largest nerve trunk of the brain stem, which may help to identify it. CN V enlarges as the trigeminal ganglion (homologous to the dorsal root ganglion of the spinal cord) before dividing into two trunks. The one that continues rostrally is the ophthalmic division or V_1, whereas the other represents the combined maxillary division or V_2 and the mandibular division or V_3. The latter trunk may divide just before or immediately after it emerges from the skull into its two separate divisions. The ophthalmic nerve enters the orbit either through the ophthalmic foramen or with the oculomotor nerve. The maxillary nerve usually emerges from the skull with the mandibular nerve through the maxillomandibular foramen.

The ophthalmic nerve transmits sensory information from the eye to the brain stem. In addition, the ophthalmic nerve has a medial branch that is sensory to the nasal cavity, hard palate, and the upper edge of the beak. It also provides the sensory information from the bill tip organ in the distal end of the upper bill or maxillary nail of geese and ducks. The lateral branch receives sensory information from the upper eyelid and skin of the forehead. A pinprick to that area of the head can be used to test for the function of V_1.

The maxillary division of CN V has three major nerve trunks. Its supraorbital nerve provides sensory innervation to the conjunctiva and skin of the dorsal eyelid. Another trunk is small in birds, the infraorbital nerve, and it supplies the lower eyelid, its conjunctiva and the skin of the rictus. The third trunk is the nasopalatine nerve. It provides sensory information from the lateral side of the beak near the cutting surface of the tomium. Additionally, fibers from CN VII or the facial nerve catch a ride on those from CN V to provide the parasympathetic innervation to the lacrimal gland and nasal glands of the nasal cavity.

The mandibular division of V (V_3) has both sensory and motor components. It innervates the muscles of mastication and those that both open and close the mouth, except for the mandibular depressor muscle. This depressor muscle is homologous to the caudal belly of the digastricus and the stylohyoideus muscles, both innervated by CN VII as in mammals. The V_3 also provides sensory information from the mandible, but its sensory supply overlaps with the maxillary nerve at the area of the rictus. A unique feature of CN V_3 in birds is that it also supplies the orbicularis oculi muscle, the muscle that closes the palpebral fissure by closing down the lid margin. This is a muscle of facial expression in mammals and is normally supplied by CN VII, but in birds, it is supplied by CN V_3. The mandibular nerve also provides sensory information from the floor of the oropharynx. In addition, fibers from CN VII hop a ride on CN V_3 and send information from taste buds in the floor of the oropharynx to the nucleus solitarius in the medulla (Fig. 5).

Abducens nerve (cranial nerve VI)

CN VI or the abducens nerve emerges ventrally from the midline of the medulla. Its nucleus is found dorsally in the rostral medulla just ventral to the fourth ventricle. The abducens nerve exits the skull through the abducent foramen and runs over the back of the eyeball. The abducens nerve supplies the extrinsic muscle to the eye, the lateral rectus muscle, and two muscles of the eyelid of the bird, the quadratus and pyramidalis muscles (see Fig. 3).

Facial nerve (cranial nerve VII)

The facial nerve exits the skull through the foramen of the facial nerve and is made up of approximately four components. One component

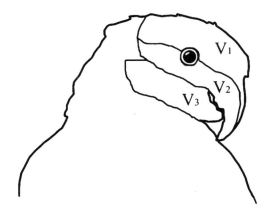

Fig. 5. Regional representation of areas served by the trigeminal nerve, cranial nerve V. Cranial nerve V forms 3 main branches. The ophthalmic nerve, V_1, receives information from the upper eyelid, the skin of the forehead, and the rostral part of the nasal cavity. The maxillary division, V_2, receives sensory information from the lower eyelid and the lateral margin of the upper bill. The mandibular division, V_3, provides motor branches to the muscles of mastication and sensory branches to the skin and mucosa at the rictus and to the lower bill. It also receives sensory information from the sensitive tip of the lower bill.

controls the muscles of facial expression; however, they are poorly developed in birds. Control of the orbicularis oculi muscle, the major facial muscle that controls eye blink, is believed to be innervated by the mandibular nerve (V_3). Another component is the muscles of mastication from CN VII. In birds, there is only one muscle innervated by CN VII, the mandibular depressor muscle. Another component of the facial nerve transmits information concerning taste from at least the tongue to the nucleus solitarius in the medulla. In many bird species, there are receptors for taste on the tongue and the mucosal lining of the oropharynx. These receptors send information to the nucleus solitarius and may be found in the floor and roof, and along the tips of the maxillary and/or mandibular bills. These sites are related to the type of bill and the food items of the particular species. Fibers from each rhamphotheca are believed to travel with components of the trigeminal nerve (see CN V), including taste fibers from the oropharynx. The fibers carrying information concerning taste, however, end in the nucleus solitarius, not the sensory nucleus of V.

The other component of CN VII supplies postganglionic parasympathetic fibers to most of the glands of the head. Birds do not have large organized salivary glands but instead have multiple microscopic ones in the epithelial lining of the oropharynx. These salivary glands are predominantly innervated by the facial nerve. Additionally, glands in the nasal mucosa, the lacrimal gland, the gland of the nictitating membrane, and nasal gland also are supplied by cranial nerve VII (see Fig. 4).

Vestibulocochlear nerve (cranial nerve VIII)

The vestibulocochlear nerve, CN VIII [30,50,62], as the name implies, has two functions (see Fig. 2). One component transmits information concerning the body in three-dimensional space from the inner ear. This information is relayed from the vestibular nuclei in the caudodorsal medulla to the cerebellum and the vestibulospinal tracts. These tracts are concerned with coordinating the body and hence posture in relation to movement of the head, and eye coordination through the medial longitudinal fasciculus (MLF). The cochlear component of CN VIII sends auditory information to basically two primary auditory nuclei in the medulla. CN VIII transits the skull through the cochlear foramen. Information is transmitted through the lateral lemniscus to the caudal colliculus for reflex control. In addition, information concerning hearing continues to the thalamus and then the telencephalon for the conscious perception of hearing.

The hearing capabilities of birds have some different characteristics compared with mammals. The ability to discriminate pitch, for example, is highly developed in some passerines and parrots. Why certain species mimic so well is not understood but most likely relates to social or environmental factors. Additionally, birds have much greater temporal resolution than mammals. Recordings of songs in passerines must be slowed down considerably in order for the human ear to pick up the details. Birds have far greater auditory localization, particularly nocturnal birds. Owls can hunt in total darkness based on their capacity to locate by sound. A small delay between sound signals from the two ears facilitates localization, a fact that may explain part of the reason that the ears of many owls are asymmetrically located. Although birds are believed to be unable to hear ultrasonic vibrations, some birds use echolocation to avoid obstacles in the dark, for example [64]. Penguins may find food in the water by echolocation also [65].

Clinically, it may be difficult to determine if the bird can hear. Birds that do not hear tend to be constantly moving their heads. A loud sound will not startle them if they are unable to pick up the sound vibrations perceived as sensory information. This information could be derived from the skin as and the specialized receptors, the interosseous membranes from Herbst corpuscles in the legs and feet [66–68]. Electrodiagnostic testing using auditory evoked potentials (AER) can be used in birds as it is in mammals (SEO and others at The University of Tennessee have performed this procedure).

Glossopharyngeal nerve (cranial nerve IX)

Cranial nerves IX, X, and XI [30,48–50,62] emerge together from the ventrolateral medulla (see Fig. 4), but emerge from the skull through different foramen. CN IX itself exits the skull through the glossopharyngeal foramen. In conjunction with CN XII, they also undergo considerable anastomoses, so that it is difficult to discriminate each of these cranial nerves on a neurological examination in birds. For example, the proximal ganglia of both cranial nerves IX and X fuse. Additionally, fibers from cranial nerves IX and X anastomose also. The lingual nerve of birds does not arise from CN V but instead is one of these anastomotic nerves. It carries sensory and taste information from the tongue. These taste fibers therefore may be from CN VII and/or cranial nerves IX and X. These combined nerves of IX and X innervate the laryngeal muscles and the overlying epithelium so that swallowing and the gag reflex are controlled by them. One anatomic difference is that the carotid body is not innervated by CN IX, as it is in mammals, but by CN X. Cranial nerves IX and X supply the crop, and, through an anastomosis with CN XII, also supply the syrinx.

Swallowing is a complex activity possibly using several of the cranial nerves as a result of the anastomoses. The gag reflex has its sensory component from CN V$_3$ and its motor component from CN IX and possibly CN X.

Vagus nerve (cranial nerve X)

The vagus nerve [30,48–50,62] is formed from multiple small rootlets from the ventrolateral medulla (see Fig. 4). They arise in concert with fibers from cranial nerves IX and XI, making it difficult to distinguish these individually on a neurological examination. CN IX may be part of the proximal ganglion, which represents a collection of cell bodies from somatic afferent fibers. The vagus nerve then dives through the vagal foramen to exit the skull. It connects with the cranial cervical ganglion and CN IX before becoming enclosed in a common sheath with CN XI. The vagus provides branches to the larynx and pharynx, most likely from its anastomoses with IX.

The distal vagal ganglion found at the thoracic inlet is composed of cell bodies from visceral afferents. In addition to supplying the carotid body, the vagus provides fibers to numerous glands of the neck including the thymus, thyroid, and parathyroid glands and the ultimobranchial bodies. A branch of the vagus, the aortic nerve, has fibers from baroreceptors in the aorta and pulmonary trunk.

The recurrent laryngeal nerve supplies the esophagus and crop. In addition, its fibers innervate the tracheal and syringeal muscles. The exact CN supply is unknown, however, because of anastomoses. The vagus provides visceral fibers to the heart and lungs. The abdominal vagus supplies the gizzard, duodenum, and liver. It usually is formed from an anastomosis of the right and left nerves to form a single trunk. It is the ganglia of the postganglionic parasympathetic fibers that are affected by the clinical condition of proventricular dilatation disease (PDD). Normal crop, stomach, and syringeal function are controlled by the vagus, and all of these components may be affected by PDD.

Accessory nerve (cranial nerve XI)

The nuclei of the accessory nerve [30,50] are found in the caudal medulla (see Fig. 4). They represent nuclei concerned with general somatic efferents to the skeletal muscles like the hypoglossal nerve. The accessory nerve in birds anastomoses with CN X. Part of this nerve branches off from the main trunk to innervate the cucularis muscle, which is homologous to the mammalian trapezius muscle. Other functions have not been described in birds. The accessory nerve emerges from the skull through the foramen magnum.

Hypoglossal nerve (cranial nerve XII)

The hypoglossal nerve [30,49,50] emerges from the ventral medulla as a small collection of rootlets (see Fig. 4). These fibers combine into approximately two nerves that travel through the skull by means of two hypoglossal canals; the exact number varies by species. After leaving the skull, they combine with the first and possibly the second cervical nerves to form the hypoglossocervical nerve. This nerve then anastomoses with cranial nerves IX and X. The nerve branches supply the tongue, tracheal, and syringeal muscles. Only psittacine birds have intrinsic muscles of the tongue. The extrinsic muscles that attach to the hypobranchial apparatus or hyoid bone allow birds tremendous mobility of their tongues. Most likely, these muscles are supplied by CN XII. Examination of cranial nerve function should include examination of the oropharynx and the tongue. The bird should be able to move the tongue if CN XII is intact. If one side is affected and non-functional, the tongue will turn toward the side of the lesion, as the muscle tone on the normal side will push it toward the side with less tone.

Summary

New integrative models of brain and behavior have positioned neuroscience centrally in the diagnosis and evaluation of avian health and care in several ways. The concept of stress provides a common currency with which the intricate relationships between a bird and diverse social and biophysical variables may be examined and assessed. Further, the discovery of homologies and homoplasies between taxa has been instrumental in bringing deeper understanding of their systems and a greater facilitation of dialog between avian and mammalian clinicians. Processes and effects of stress on psychobiology, and hence diagnosis and treatment, may be complex, but by bringing awareness of their importance, a more comprehensive foundation for avian care is possible.

References

[1] Jarvis E, Gunturkun O, Bruce L, et al. Avian brains and a new understanding of vertebrate brain evolution. Nat Rev Neurosci 2005;6(2):151–9.
[2] Pepperberg IM. The Alex studies: cognitive and communicative abilities of grey parrots. Harvard (IL): Harvard University Press; 2000.
[3] Emery NJ, Clayton NS. Comparing the complex cognition of birds and primates. In: Rogers LJ, Kaplan G, editors. Comparative vertebrate cognition. Norwell (MA): Kluwer Academic/Plenum; 2004. p. 3–56.
[4] Emery NJ, Clayton NS. Effects of experience and social context on prospective caching strategies by scrub jays. Nature 2004;414(6832):443–6.
[5] Dally JM, Emery NJ, Clayton NS. Food-caching Western scrub jays keep track of who was watching when. Science 2006;312(5780):1662–5.
[6] Groothuis TG, Carere C. Avian personalities: characterization and epigenesis. Neurosci Biobehav Rev 2005;29(1):137–50.
[7] Prather JF, Mooney R. Neural correlates of learned song in the avian forebrain: simultaneous representation for self and others. Curr Opin Neurobiol 2004;14(4):496–502.
[8] Chappell J, Kacelnik A. Tool selectivity in a nonmammal, the New Caledonian crow (*Corvus moneduloides*). Anim Cogn 2002;5(2):71–8.
[9] Haesler SK, Wada A, Nshdejan EE, et al. *FoxP2* expression in avian vocal learners and non-learners. J Neurosci 2004;24(13):3164–75.
[10] Panksepp J. Affective neurosciences: the foundations of human and animal emotions. Oxford (OH): Oxford University Press; 1998.
[11] Emery NJ. Are corvids feathered apes? Cognitive evolution in crows, jays, rooks, and jackdaws. In: Watanabe S, editor. Comparative analysis of minds. Tokyo: Keio University Press; 2004. p. 181–213.

[12] Davidson RJ, Scherer KR, Hill Goldsmith H, editors. Handbook of affective sciences. Oxford (OH): Oxford University Press; 2004.

[13] LeDoux J. The emotional brain: the mysterious underpinnings of emotional life. New York: Touchstone Books; 1996.

[14] Goleman D. Social intelligence: the new science of human relationships. New York: Bantam Books; 2006.

[15] Berridge KC. Comparing the emotional brains of humans and other animals. In: Davidson RJ, Scherer KR, Hill Goldsmith H, editors. Handbook of affective sciences. Oxford (OH): Oxford University Press; 2003. p. 23–45.

[16] Bradshaw GA, Sapolsky RM. Mirror, mirror. Am Sci 2006;94(6):487–9.

[17] Orosz SE. Principles of avian clinical neuroanatomy. Seminars in Avian and Exotic Pet Medicine 1996;5(3):127–39.

[18] Boonstra R. Coping with changing northern environment: the role of the stress axis in birds and mammals. Integr Comp Biol 2004;44(2):85–108.

[19] Sapolsky RM. Why zebras don't get ulcers: a guide to stress, stress-related disease, and coping. 3rd edition. New York: Owl Books; 2004.

[20] Buwalda B, Kole MH, Veenema AH, et al. Long-term effects of social stress on brain and behavior: a focus on hippocampal functioning. Neurosci Biobehav Rev 2005;29(11):83–97.

[21] van der Kolk BA, McFarlane AC, Weisaeth L. Traumatic stress; the effects of overwhelming experience on mind, body, and society. London: Guilford Press; 1996.

[22] Bartolomucci A, Palanza P, Sacerdote P, et al. Social factors and individual vulnerability to chronic stress exposure. Neurosci Biobehav Rev 2005;29(1):67–81.

[23] West MJ, King AP, White DJ. The case for developmental ecology. Anim Behav 2003;66(4): 617–22.

[24] Goldstein MH, King AP, West MJ. Social interaction shapes babbling: testing parallels between birdsong and speech. Proc Natl Acad Sci U S A 2003;100(13):8030–5.

[25] Siegel DJ. The developing mind: toward a neurobiology of interpersonal experience. New York: Guilford Press; 1999.

[26] Suomi SJ. How gene–environment interactions can influence emotional development in rhesus monkeys. In: Garcia-Coll CE, Bearer L, Lerner RM, editors. Nature and nurture: the complex interplay of genetic and environmental influences on human behavior and development. Mahwah (NJ): Lawrence Erlbaum; 2004. p. 35–51.

[27] Meaney MJ. Maternal care, gene expression, and the transmission of individual differences in stress reactivity across generations. Annu Rev Neurosci 2001;24:1161–92.

[28] Meaney MJ, Szyf M. Maternal care as a model for experience-dependent chromatin plasticity? Trends Neurosci 2005;28(9):456–63.

[29] Walker B, Wingfeild JC, Dee Boersma P. Age and food deprivation affects expression of the glucocorticosteroid stress response in Magellanic penguin (Spheniscus magellanicus) chicks. Physiol Biochem Zool 2005;78(1):78–89.

[30] King AS, McClelland J. Birds: their structure and function. 2nd edition. Bath (United Kingdom): Bailliere Tindall; 1984.

[31] Orosz SE, Delaney CJ. Self-injurious behavior (SIB) of primates as a model for feather damaging behavior (FDB) in companion psittacine birds. Proceedings of the Annual Conference of the Association of Avian Veterinarians 2003;39–50.

[32] Schore AN. Affect dysregulation and disorders of the self. New York: W.W. Norton; 2003.

[33] Curley JP, Keverne EP. Genes, brains, and mammalian social bonds. Trends Ecol Evol 2005; 2(10):561–7.

[34] Insel TR. A neurobiological basis of attachment. Am J Psychiatry 1997;154(6):726–35.

[35] Sims CG, Holberton RL. Development of the corticosterone stress response in young northern mockingbirds (Mimus polyglottos). Gen Comp Endocrinol 2000;119(2):193–201.

[36] Ladd CO, Huot RL, Thrivikraman KV, et al. Long-term adaptations in glucocorticoid receptor and mineralocorticoid receptor mRNA and negative feedback on the hypoathalamo-pituitary-adrenal axis following maternal separation. Biological Psychology 2004;55(4):367–75.

[37] Garner JP, Meehan CL, Mensch JA. Stereotypies in caged parrots, schizophrenia and autism: evidence for a common mechanism. Behav Brain Res 2003;145(1-2):125–34.

[38] Wiedenmayer CP. Adaptations or pathologies? Long-term changes in brain and behavior after a single exposure to severe threat. Neurosci Biobehav Rev 2004;28(1):1–12.

[39] Cirulli F, Berry A, Alleva E. Early disruption of the mother–infant relationship: effects on brain plasticity and implications for psychopathology. Neurosci Biobehav Rev 2003; 27(1-2):73–82.

[40] Fox RA. Hand rearing: behavioral impacts and implications for captive parrot welfare. In: Leuscher AU, editor. Manual of parrot behavior. Ames (IA): Blackwell; 2006. p. 83–92.

[41] Siebert L. Social behavior in psittacine birds. In: Leuscher AU, editor. Manual of parrot behavior. Ames (IA): Blackwell; 2006. p. 43–8.

[42] Romagnano A. Mate trauma. In: Leuscher AU, editor. Manual of parrot behavior. Ames (IA): Blackwell; 2006. p. 247–54.

[43] Herman J. Trauma and recovery. New York: Basic Books; 1997.

[44] Linden PG, Leuscher AU. 2006 Behavioral development of psittacine companion neonates, neophytes, and fledglings. In: Leuscher AU, editor. Manual of parrot behavior. Ames (IA): Blackwell; 2006. p. 93–112.

[45] Sturkie PD, editor. Avian physiology. 4th edition. New York: Springer Verlag; 1976. p. 1–73.

[46] Pessacq Asenjo TP. The nerve endings of the glycogen body of embryonic and adult spinal cord: on the existence of two different varieties of nerve fibers. Growth 1984;48(3): 385–90.

[47] Baumel JJ. Suspensory ligaments of nerves: an adaptation for protection of the avian spinal cord. Zentralblatt fur Veterinarmedizin Reihe C: Anatomia Histologia Embryologia 1985; 14(1):1–5.

[48] Carpenter MB. Core text of neuroanatomy. 2nd edition. Baltimore (MD): Williams & Wilkin; 1978.

[49] De Lahunta A, editor. Veterinary neuroanatomy and clinical neurology. Philadelphia: WB Saunders; 1977. p. 89–160.

[50] Breazile JE, Kvenzel WJ. Systema nervosum centrale. In: Baumel JJ, editor. Handbook of avian anatomy: *Nomina anatomica avium*. Cambridge (MA): Nuttall Ornithological Club; No. 23; 1993. p. 493–554.

[51] Miller L. Some tagging experiments with black-footed albatrosses. Condor 1942;44:3–9.

[52] Balthazart J, Schoffeniels E. Pheromones are involved in the control of sexual behavior in birds. Naturwissenschaften 1979;66(1):55–6.

[53] Cohen J. Olfaction and parental behavior in ring doves. Biochem Syst Ecol 1981;9:351–4.

[54] Clark L, Mason JR. Use of nest material as insecticidal and antipathogenic agents by the European starling. Oecologia 1985;67(22):169–76.

[55] Clark L, Mason JR. Olfactory discrimination of plant volatiles by the European starling. Anim Behav 1987;35(11):227–35.

[56] Clark L, Mason JR. Effect of biologically active plants used as nest material and the derived benefit to starling nestlings. Oecologia 1988;77:174–80.

[57] Clark L. The nest protection hypothesis: the adaptive use of plant secondary compounds by European starlings. In: Loye JE, Zuk B, editors. Bird–parasite interactions: ecology, evolution, and behavior. Oxford (OH): Oxford Univ. Press; 1991. p. 205–21.

[58] Tucker D, Graziadei PC, Smith JC. Recovery of olfactory function in pigeons after bilateral transaction of the olfactory nerves. In: Denton DA, Coghlan JP, editors. Olfaction and taste. New York: Academic Press; 1974. p. 369–73.

[59] Tucker D. Nonolfactory responses from the nasal cavity: Jacobson's organ and the trigeminal system. In: Beidler LM, editor. Handbook of sensory physiology IV: chemical senses, olfaction. Berlin: Springer-Verlag; 1971. p. 151–81.

[60] Gunturkun O. Sensory physiology: vision. In: Whittow GC, editor. Sturkie's avian physiology. 5th edition. San Diego (CA): Academic Press; 2000. p. 1–19.

[61] Rogers JJ, Miles FA. Centrifugal control of the avian retina. V. Effects of lesions of the isthmo-optic nucleus on visual behaviour. Brain Res 1972;48:147–56.

[62] Szekely G, Matesz C, et al. The efferent system of cranial nerve nuclei: a comparative neuromorphological study. In: Beck F, Hild W, Kriz W, editors. Advances in anatomy, embryology and cell biology. Vol. 128. New York: Springer Verlag; 1993. p. 1–79.

[63] Portman A, Stingelin W. The central nervous system. In: Marshal AJ, editor. Biology and comparative physiology of birds Vol. II. New York: Academic Press; 1961. p. 1–36.

[64] Necker R. The avian ear and hearing. In: Whittow GC, editor. Sturkie's avian physiology. 5th edition. San Diego (CA): Academic Press; 2000. p. 21–38.

[65] Poulter TC. Sonar of penguins and fur seals. Proceedings of the California Academy of Sciences. 1969;36:363–80.

[66] Orosz SE. The special senses of birds. In: Coles B, editor. Essentials of avian medicine and surgery. 3rd edition. Oxford (OH): Blackwell Publishing; 2007. in press.

[67] Schildmacher H. Untersuchungen über die Funktion der Kerbstchen Körperchen. J Ornithol 1931;79:374–415.

[68] Schwartzkopff J. Über Sitz und Leistung von Gehör und Vibrationssinn bei Vögeln. Zeitschrift fuer Vergleichende Physiologie 1949;31:527–608.

ELSEVIER
SAUNDERS

VETERINARY
CLINICS
Exotic Animal Practice

Vet Clin Exot Anim 10 (2007) 803–836

The Avian Neurologic Examination and Ancillary Neurodiagnostic Techniques: A Review Update

Tracy L. Clippinger, DVM, DACZM[a],*,
R. Avery Bennett, DVM, MS, DACVS[b],
Simon R. Platt, BVMS, MCRVS,
DACVIM, DECVN[c]

[a]Department of Veterinary Services, Zoological Society of San Diego-San Diego Zoo,
1354 Old Globe Way, San Diego, CA 92101-1635, USA
[b]Department of Veterinary Clinical Medicine, College of Veterinary Medicine,
University of Illinois, 1008 West Hazelwood Drive, Urbana, IL 61802, USA
[c]Department of Small Animal Medicine and Surgery, College of Veterinary Medicine,
University of Georgia, 501 DW Brooks Drive Athens, GA 30602-7371, USA

An understanding of basic avian neuroanatomy and physiology is necessary to evaluate abnormal function of the nervous system [1–10]. A complete neurologic examination is necessary to localize the anatomic distribution of neurologic disease, to determine the severity of dysfunction, and to assess the prognosis for patient recovery. The findings of the history, physical examination, basic neurologic examination, and minimum database guide the need for and use of survey radiography, cerebrospinal fluid (CSF) analysis, diagnostic imaging, electrodiagnostics, and histopathology. Once the disease location and pathologic process have been identified, appropriate treatment and prognosis may be provided.

Neurologic examination

A neurologic examination [11–18] is integrated easily into a routine physical examination and may be recorded by a simple format adapted for use in avian patients (Fig. 1).

Modified with permission from: Clippinger TL, Bennett RA, Platt SR. The Avian Neurologic Examination and Ancillary Neurodiagnostic Techniques. J Av Med Surg 1996;10(4):221–47.
* Corresponding author.
E-mail address: tclippinger@sandiegozoo.org (T.L. Clippinger).

doi:10.1016/j.cvex.2007.04.006

AVIAN NEUROLOGIC EXAMINATION

Patient_____   Date & Time_____

Species_____   Age_____   Sex_____

SUBJECTIVE:

OBJECTIVE:
Observation
    Mentation: _____
    alert, depression, stupor, coma, delirium
    Posture: _____
    normal, recumbency, opisthotonos
    Attitude: _____
    normal, strabismus, head tilt, falling
    Movement: _____
    normal, spasm, tremble, twitch, seizure
    Gait: _____
    normal, ataxia, dysmetria, circling, weakness
Cranial Nerve Reflexes

L	*nerve, test*	R
	I	
	odor	
	II & V	
	menace	
	II & III	
	direct PLR	
	III, IV, VI	
	strabismus	
	III, IV, VI, VIII	
	nystagmus	
	V	
	palpebral, sensation	
	VII	
	expression	
	VIII	
	startle, balance	
	IX	
	bitter taste	
	IX, X, XI, XII	
	gag , visceral	
	XII	
	tongue grab	

OBJECTIVE:
Palpation
Muscle/Skeleton_____
    symmetry, tone, strength, tenderness
Postural reactions
    L   *reaction*   R
    Conscious proprioception
    _____ wings _____
    _____ legs _____
    Drop and flap
    _____ wings _____
    Hopping
    _____ legs _____
    Extensor postural thrust
    _____ legs _____
    Tactile Placing
    _____ legs _____
    Visual Placing
    _____ legs _____
Spinal Reflexes

L	*reflex, segment*	R
	Vent sphincter	
	LSP-P & LSP-Cd	
	Leg withdrawal	
	LSP-S	
	Patella	
	LSP-L	
	Wing withdrawal	
	BP	

Sensory response
    _____pelvic
    _____thoracic
    hyperesthesia, superficial pain, deep pain

ASSESSMENT: localizing deficits
•Normal
•Brain
    Cerebrum_____
    Cerebellum_____
    Brain stem_____
    Vestibular_____

•Spinal cord
    Cervical_____
    Brachial plexus _____
    Thoracic_____
    Lumbosacral plexus_____
•Peripheral nerve_____
•Generalized neuromuscular_____

PLAN: Recommended tests   Differential diagnosis:

Fig. 1. A sample form for recording findings of the avian neurologic examination is presented. Diagrams of the location of the cranial nerve roots and the brain regions are included. (*From* Clippinger TL, Bennett RA, Platt SR. The avian neurologic examination and ancillary neurodiagnostic techniques. J Av Med Surg 1996;10(4):221–47; with permission).

Observation of the bird allows evaluation of mentation, posture, attitude, and gait. Changes in mentation (level and content of consciousness) are revealed by a history of personality change, change in awareness of surroundings, and inappropriate behavioral responses to situations. Obtundation, stupor, and coma are changes in the level of consciousness and indicate functional damage to pathways mediated through the brain stem (arousal) or diffuse damage to the cerebral cortex (content and regulation) [14]. Metabolic or systemic disorders that render a bird ill generally cause depression and lethargy. Confusion, dementia, and delirium are changes in the content of consciousness and indicate structural or metabolic damage to the cerebrum [14].

Posture is the position of the body with respect to gravity, and it requires the limbs to act as antigravity support columns. Neurologic maintenance of erect posture requires interaction between sensory receptors and motor activators in the peripheral nervous system (PNS) and integration by pathways in the central nervous system (CNS). Recumbency may result from lethargy (systemic illness), extreme pain, or neurologic dysfunction (pathologic process). Losses of muscle power or flaccidity are lower motor neuron signs and indicate a lesion in the nerve connecting the affected muscle to the CNS. Increased muscle tone or rigidity are upper motor neuron signs and indicate a lesion in the CNS cranial to the affected anatomic section [14]. A lesion within the rostral brain stem may cause a comatose state and decerebrate rigidity. Opisthotonus indicates damage to the cerebellum or to the brainstem [14].

Attitude, a component of posture, is the position of the eyes, head, and limbs with respect to the body. The vestibular system has central (cerebellum, brain stem, spinal cord) and peripheral elements (labyrinth of the inner ear and vestibulocochlear nerve) that are responsible for attitude. Central lesions receive normal peripheral input but scramble the output; peripheral lesions change input so the central system attempts to make adjustments to maintain attitude. This central correcting response often is preserved so that abnormalities are observed on the diseased side of the body. Nystagmus, head tilt, leaning, falling, and compulsive rolling or circling are signs of altered attitude. Positional nystagmus in association with changes in mentation and changes in proprioception indicate central disease [14]. Peripheral disease generally produces spontaneous horizontal nystagmus, a head tilt in the acute stage, and a tendency for tight circling [14]. The wide-based stance of a resting bird on a perch may reflect injury to the vestibular system [1], although a wide-based stance may be seen in all forms of ataxia and in cases of generalized weakness [14].

Movement and gait describe the ability of the patient to perform normal activities, and patients should be evaluated for coordination and strength in both voluntary and involuntary motion. Coordinated voluntary limb movements require functional cerebral, cerebellar, vestibular, and proprioceptive pathways. Lack of precise or finely tuned movement indicates a lesion in the cerebrum [14]. Birds with cerebral disease may be able to walk, but may not be able to step up and over or onto different sized branches. Limb movements that are excessive or deficient signal cerebellar disease. Leaning or falling and loss of balance indicate damage to the vestibular system. Weak or absent voluntary limb movements (paresis or plegia) suggest disruption of pathways that run through the cerebral cortex, brain stem, spinal cord, and the peripheral nerves.

Involuntary limb and body motion such as tremors and seizures are common clinical signs associated with primary or secondary damage to the brain [19]. A bird that uncontrollably shakes its head as it approaches the food bowl has intention tremors, a sign of cerebellar disease. Seizures result from spontaneous bursts of neuronal activity in the cerebral cortex. Clinical signs ranging from focal muscle activity to tonic–clonic convulsions help determine the location or generalization of the seizure focus in the cerebrum [12]. In addition to intracranial disease [19–28], seizures and tremors also may result from extracranial influences [1,19,29] on the cerebral cortex, including metabolic disturbances [30], parasite migration or presence [31–37], toxic disorders [38–51], and nutritional deficiencies [30,52,53].

Cranial nerves

Evaluation of the cranial nerves (CNs) follows assessment of the head and face for attitude and symmetry. Because each cranial nerve exits the brain at a distinct location, the cranial nerve examination serves a vital role in localizing damage to specific regions of the brain. Several reflexes evaluated in the cranial nerve examination require separate intact sensory and motor nerves, potentially allowing more precise lesion localization. All 12 cranial nerves should be evaluated in sequence beginning with the most rostral before attempting to make conclusions. Some differences exist between the neuroanatomy of avian and mammalian species [1,2,4,7–9,16,54–56]. CN function, testing, and signs of dysfunction are summarized in Table 1.

Disorders in olfaction (CN I) may be suggested in the history by altered appetite and feeding behaviors, but are difficult to evaluate objectively.

Ophthalmic examination helps identify problems in optic (CN II), oculomotor (CN III), trochlear (CN IV), abducens (CN VI), and trigeminal (CN V) nerves [2,4,7,8,10,55,56]. The ability to avoid obstacles indicates integrity of the optic nerve and cerebral pathways. The menace response is a learned response that is initiated by the cerebrum whenever a threat is perceived. The menace response in birds requires an intact CN II to see a potential threat and an intact CN V (orbicularis oculi muscle) to protect the eye by eyelid closure [8,10,55]. Birds that are stoic or very excited may not show a menace response even though nerve function is intact. Shining a bright light directly into the eye of a normal bird causes constriction of the pupil. The light is sensed by CN II; parasympathetic fibers of CN III cause contraction of the iris muscle (miosis). Birds have striated muscle in the iris, giving them some voluntary control over pupil size independent of light intensity. The pupillary light response (PLR) is evaluated best early in the examination, as sympathetic tone in restrained birds may override constriction. Some birds have an incomplete bony septum between the globes and may respond to light reaching the contralateral retina, mimicking a consensual response. In a recent study in chicks, transection of the optic nerve allowed confirmation of an indirect PLR in the absence of a direct PLR and demonstrated a direct, but no indirect, PLR response in the non-operated eye [57]. Cranial nerves III, IV, and VI aid vision by maintaining the globe in a central position. Deviation of the globe from its central axis indicates dysfunction in one or more of these nerves: ventrolateral deviation (CN III), dorsolateral deviation (CN IV), and medial deviation (CN VI). In contrast to mammals, the third eyelid in birds has striated muscle fibers innervated by CN VI that initiate movement of the nictitans across the cornea [8,10,12,55,58]. Prolapse of the third eyelid in birds may indicate loss of sympathetic innervation as found in Horner's syndrome in mammals [59,60].

The trigeminal nerve (CN V) is responsible for facial sensation, while the motor response to facial sensory stimulation is generally provided by the facial nerve (CN VII). The eyelids are completely innervated by CN V in birds [4,7,8,55]. Eyelid sensation is provided by its ophthalmic branch (upper lid) and its maxillary branch (both lids). Eyelid closure is provided by its mandibular branch (orbicularis oculi muscle). Touching the medial canthus of the normal eyelid elicits lid closure. The mandibular branch of CN V also provides motor function to the jaw [4,8]. A dropped lower beak or the inability to chew indicates damage to CN V. Cranial nerve VII contributes to prehension by partial innervation of the muscles that open the jaw. Cranial nerve VII maintains facial symmetry, however the facial musculature in birds is minimal, making evaluation difficult. Most of the glands of the head receive parasympathetic innervation from CN VII, so decreased secretions may indicate damage to that nerve. Sensory innervation to the lingual taste buds is shared by CN VII and the glossopharyngeal nerve (CN IX).

The vestibulochlear nerve (CN VIII) is involved in sensory perception of noise and in maintaining equilibrium. Evidence of hearing and thus, integrity of the cochlear branch of CN VIII, may be challenging to assess in birds. Balance is maintained by the vestibular system, which has central elements in the brain and spinal cord, and peripheral elements in the inner ear (semicircular canal labyrinth apparatus) and CN VIII. The vestibular system keeps the limbs positioned to support the body, the head upright, and the eyes fixed on objects in a horizontal plane. Moving the head from side to side in a horizontal plane induces physiologic nystagmus with the fast phase in the direction of head movement. This oculocephalic reflex tests the integrity of CN VIII (sensory), and CN III, IV, and VI (motor). Clinical signs of peripheral vestibular disease manifest after damage to the inner ear or vestibular branch of CN VIII that effectively gives unbalanced input to the intact central vestibular system [12]. In the absence of head motion, spontaneous horizontal nystagmus is consistent with CN VIII damage with the fast component away from the side of the lesion. Unilateral peripheral vestibular disease may cause a head tilt and circling toward the affected side. Positional nystagmus in association with changes in mentation and changes in proprioception indicate central disease.

Table 1
The function, means of testing, and clinical signs of dysfunction of the cranial nerves in birds

	Nerve	Function	Test	Signs of dysfunction
I	Olfactory	Sensory—smell	Odor	Impaired smell
II	Optic	Sensory—vision	Menace	Impaired sight
III	Oculomotor	Motor—extrinsic ocular muscle	Eyeball position	Ventrolateral deviation
		Upper eyelid muscle	Menace	Drooped upper eyelid
		Parasympathetic—intrinsic ocular muscle	Pupillary light reflex	Dilated pupil
IV	Trochlear	Motor—extrinsic ocular muscle	Eyeball position	Dorsolateral deviation
V	Trigeminal	Sensory—ophthalmic branch (upper lid, forehead skin, nasal cavity, upper beak)	Skin touch	Facial hypesthesia
		Sensory—maxillary branch (both lids, hard palate, nasal cavity, lateral upper beak)	Palpebral	
		Motor—mandibular branch (orbicularis, lower lid, chewing)	Palpebral	Wide palpebral fissure
		Sensory – mandibular branch (lower beak skin commissures)	Pinch jaw	Unable to close jaw
VI	Abducens	Motor—extrinsic ocular muscle	Eyeball position	Medial deviation
		Third eyelid muscle		Third eyelid immobility
VII	Facial	Motor—facial expression		Asymmetry of face
		Sensory—taste		Poor taste
		Parasympathetic—most glands of head		Decreased secretions

CN	Nerve	Function	Test/Reflex	Clinical signs
VIII	Vestibulo–cochlear	Sensory—hearing	Startle	Impaired hearing
		Sensory—balance and coordination	Oculocephalic	Nystagmus, head tilt
IX[a]	Glosso–pharyngeal	Sensory—tongue sense and taste, trachea		Poor taste and feel
		Motor-pharynx, larynx, crop, syrinx	Gag reflex	Dysphagia, voice loss
X[a]	Vagus	Sensory—larynx, pharynx, viscera	Gag reflex	Regurgitation
		Motor—larynx, pharynx, esophagus, crop		Voice change
		Parasympathetic—to glands, viscera	Oculo-cardiac	Increased heart rate / No crop motility
XI[a]	Accessory	Motor—superficial neck muscles		Poor neck movement
XII[a]	Hypoglossal	Motor—tongue, trachea, syrinx	Tongue grab	Tongue deviation

[a] Anastomosis present involving cranial nerves IX–XII.

From Clippinger TL, Bennett RA, Platt SR. The Avian Neurologic Examination and Ancillary Neurodiagnostic Techniques. J Av Med Surg 1996;10(4):221–47; with permission.

The remaining four cranial nerves have variable origins and significant anastomoses between distal nerve fibers in birds [4,8,55,56], making distinction of specific nerve involvement difficult. Dysphagia and regurgitation could indicate an abnormality in any or all of the last four CNs [61]. In general, lingual disorders point to a lesion of the glossopharyngeal nerve (CN IX), the hypoglossal nerve (CN XII), or both. Deviation and decreased tone of the tongue indicate injury to CN XII. Visceral signs in the cranial gastrointestinal tract (lack of rhythmic contractions) and the heart (increased rate) associated with parasympathetic dysfunction suggest disorders in the vagus nerve (CN X), the spinal accessory nerve (CN XI), or both.

Palpation

The skin, skeleton, and muscles are palpated and assessed for symmetry, masses, tenderness, contour, tone, and strength. The vertebral column should be palpated for deviations. Unilateral muscle atrophy or paresis may indicate disuse or lower motor neuron disease. Increased muscle tone may indicate upper motor neuron disease.

Postural reactions

The postural reactions require intact sensory and motor pathways throughout the nervous system and unimpaired processing and integration in the brain. Their complexity allows detection of minor deficits in any key component of the pathway. Deficits are seen caudal to or at the level of a lesion [12,14]. Postural reactions reflect the patient's ability to respond to stimuli to keep the body upright. Postural reactions require input from both the PNS, which adjusts muscle tone to prevent collapse and maintain balance, and the CNS, which coordinates and smoothes movement [14]. To test a postural reaction, a wing or leg is placed in an abnormal position, and a correcting response to fold the wings and to place the legs hip-width apart is observed.

Conscious proprioception is the patient's awareness of limb position and movement without visual information. The sensory branch of proprioception is carried from the skin of the leg through the spinal cord and brain stem to the sensorimotor cortex, where the brain responds by sending messages back to the lower motor neuron for motor function resulting in correcting the foot placement [12,18]. Ascending sensory pathways are located in the outermost regions of the spinal cord and are very sensitive to compression [8,12,14]. Placing the bird's foot on its dorsal surface against a perch and noting the bird's ability to place the foot around the perch tests this pathway. Alternatively, a sheet of paper or similar material may be placed under each foot and slowly moved sideways to see if the bird returns its foot to the standing position. A bird standing on its knuckles has proprioceptive deficits. Pulling the bird's wing away from its body and evaluating its ability to return the wing to a normal, folded position ready for takeoff crudely tests this pathway in the thoracic limbs.

Hopping requires one limb to compensate for the loss of the other limb and to carry the full weight of the body when the patient is moved forward and from side to side. Bandaging or holding one leg up against the body forces the bird to support weight on one limb. Unfortunately, most birds do not tolerate restraint in this manner and will focus on biting the handler or escaping. Pushing the bird to the side and evaluating the compensatory response of the limb opposite the side to which the force is applied tests the same pathway as the hopping reaction. Poor initiation suggests sensory deficits, whereas poor follow-through suggests motor deficits [14].

The drop and flap reaction tests the response of the thoracic limbs to loss of body support. The legs are grasped close to the body, the bird is held high, and a simulated drop is performed. The bird also may be dropped onto a soft cushion. The bird should pull equally with both wings to prevent its fall to the ground. The simulated drop may be adjusted to either side, and the down wing should flap harder to compensate for a fall to that side. Slow initiation supports a lesion in the cervical spinal cord, the brain stem, or the cerebral cortex [14].

The extensor postural thrust reaction is elicited by holding the bird around the body and wings and lowering it to the ground. The pelvic limbs should move in a walking fashion to achieve a support position for the body. As with the drop and flap reaction, this test evaluates ascending sensory pathways to the cerebral cortex and descending motor pathways to the limb.

Placing reactions of the wings and the tonic neck reaction are not evaluated routinely in birds. Placing reactions of the rear limbs may be helpful in certain cases. Visual placing may be evaluated crudely by offering a perch for the patient to step onto. Tactile placing may be evaluated in birds that allow blindfolding, such as raptors and ratites. A perch may be touched to the dorsum of each foot to initiate a step-up. Hooded ratites may be led up to a small step or curb to test placement. Both visual and tactile placing reactions require intact motor cortex and motor pathways to the involved limb. Visual placing requires sensation from the eyes (CN II) and transmission through the visual cortex, whereas tactile placing requires sensation from the skin and transmission through the spinal cord.

Spinal reflexes

Spinal (segmental) reflexes evaluate the integrity of reflex arcs and any influence from the brain on the reflex arc. Completion of a reflex requires an intact sensory nerve that provides transmission to the spinal cord and an intact motor nerve that elicits function from the innervated muscle. The reflex arc itself does not involve the brain or the remainder of the spinal cord. The brain may modulate reflex activity through its ascending and descending pathways. Lesions in the motor arm of the reflex arc, termed lower motor neuron (LMN), may cause a hyporeflexia or areflexia. Hyper-reflexia results from an interruption in descending motor pathways that modulate the reflex, termed upper motor neuron (UMN).

Unlike mammals, the number of spinal nerves in birds varies with species, from 38 in pigeons to 51 in ostriches [8,54,55]. Each vertebral segment has an associated pair of spinal nerves, formed by a small dorsal root (sensory) and a large ventral root (motor) arising from the spinal cord. The brachial plexus, made up of branches of four to five spinal nerves, innervates the thoracic body wall and wings [4,54,55]. Made up of eight or more spinal nerves and embedded in the foveae of the synsacrum, the lumbosacral plexus contains the lumbar plexus, sacral plexus, and pudendal plexus [4,7,54,55] and innervates the caudal abdominal body wall, legs, vent, and tail [4,55]. The lumbosacral plexus is situated near or within the kidney, so that renal distortion may affect portions of the plexus [1,55].

The spinal cord enlargements divide the cord with its spinal nerves into major regions for evaluation: cervical region, brachial plexus, thoracic region, and lumbosacral plexus. The integrity of each spinal cord region is reflected in the tone and movement of muscles caudal to the region: tail–caudal spinal nerves and pudendal plexus, vent sphincter and cloaca–pudendal plexus, leg–sacral plexus and lumbar plexus, and wing–brachial plexus. Spinal reflexes and lower motor neuron/upper motor neuron signs in the limbs help to localize lesions to regions of the spinal cord (Fig. 2).

A relaxed, laterally recumbent, minimally restrained patient is a prerequisite for evaluating spinal reflexes. This situation is often difficult to obtain with avian patients.

The vent sphincter reflex gives information regarding the pudendal plexus and caudal segments of the spinal cord. Pinching or pricking the vent in a normal bird causes a wink-like contraction of the external sphincter muscles and a tail bob. A flaccid vent and overdistended cloaca that is expressed easily indicate lower motor neuron damage to the pudendal nerve or its spinal roots. A hypertonic vent indicates upper motor neuron damage at any point craniad to the pudendal plexus.

The pedal flexor reflex, a withdrawal reflex, elicits contraction of flexor muscle groups in the leg in response to a pinch stimulus to the skin of the foot. Presence of the withdrawal reflex requires an intact ischiatic nerve (sensory and motor) and an intact spinal segment at the sacral plexus, but does not require transmission along the spinal cord to the brain. Absence of the withdrawal reflex in the leg denotes extensive lower motor neuron damage involving the sacral plexus or the ischiatic nerve. A space-occupying mass within the kidney or pelvic canal, such as a renal tumor or an egg, may impinge upon the lumbosacral plexus and its nerve, causing a hyporeflexic or areflexic withdrawal in the legs [1,62].

The contralateral limb is monitored during assessment of the pedal withdrawal reflex. Extension of the contralateral limb during flexion of the

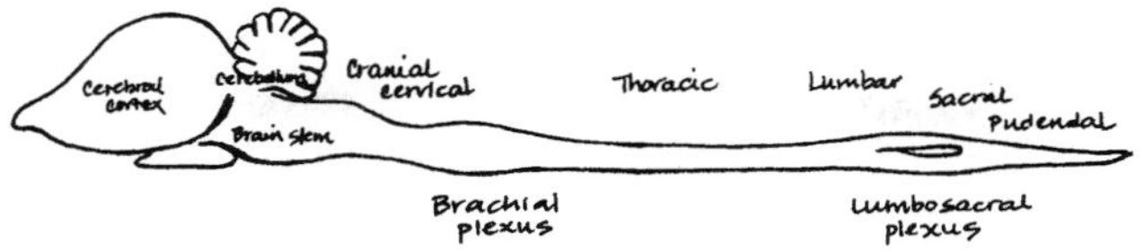

Spinal cord region	Reflexes and signs
Cranial cervical region	No cranial nerve deficits
	UMN[a] wing
	UMN leg
	UMN vent
Brachial plexus	No head signs
	LMN[b] wing
	UMN leg
	UMN vent
Peripheral nerve of wing	No head signs
	LMN wing
	No leg signs
	No vent signs
Thoracic region	No head signs
	No wing signs
	UMN leg
	UMN vent
Lumbosacral plexus (lumbar and sacral)	No head signs
	No wing signs
	LMN leg
	LMN vent
Peripheral nerve of leg	No head signs
	No wing signs
	LMN leg
	No vent signs
Lumbosacral plexus (pudendal)	No head signs
	No wing signs
	No leg signs
	LMN vent

[a] UMN = Upper motor neuron.
[b] LMN = Lower motor neuron.

Fig. 2. Localization of lesions in birds to spinal cord regions by evaluation of spinal cord reflexes and presence of upper or lower motor neuron signs. (*From* Clippinger TL, Bennett RA, Platt SR. The avian neurologic examination and ancillary neurodiagnostic techniques. J Av Med Surg 1996;10(4):221–47; with permission.)

stimulated limb denotes a positive crossed extensor reflex. In recumbent animals, descending pathways through the spinal cord inhibit extension of the contralateral limb, a normal postural response for weight-bearing standing animals [12,14]. The crossed extensor reflex indicates an upper motor neuron disease cranial to the tested limb. Presence of crossed extension in a leg denotes damage to the spinal cord cranial to the lumbosacral plexus.

The patellar reflex, a myotactic (stretch) reflex, evaluates a tap stimulus to the straight patellar tendon that effectively stretches the femorotibialis muscle [63]. This stretch stimulates the femoral nerve (lumbosacral plexus), which generates contraction of the femorotibialis muscle to extend the stifle. Certain birds, such as ostriches [64], do not have a patella; the homologous straight quadriceps tendon is stimulated. Plexor size must be adapted to patient size for improved accuracy. Because the skin associated with the inguinal web sometimes restricts the ability to isolate the stifle, this reflex may be difficult to elicit in birds. Brain or spinal cord lesions cranial to the lumbosacral plexus (upper motor neuron) cause hyper-reflexia. Upper motor neuron disease also should be accompanied by paresis [14]. Disease in the lumbosacral plexus or peripheral muscle or nerve (lower motor neuron) causes hyporeflexia. The gastrocnemius reflex is a less reliable reflex testing the tibial branch of the ischiatic nerve. Striking the gastrocnemius tendon generates extension of the hock.

The wing withdrawal reflex also should be evaluated to test the integrity of the reflex arc to the brachial plexus spinal segment. A pinch stimulus to the major digit at the leading edge of the primary flight feathers generates flexion of the wing. Absence of the withdrawal reflex in a wing indicates damage to the brachial plexus or its nerves. A positive crossed extensor reflex of a wing denotes damage cranial to the brachial plexus within the cervical spinal cord or the brain stem (upper motor neuron).

Cutaneous sensation

Done at the end of the neurologic examination to avoid losing patient co-operation, testing of cutaneous sensation provides information regarding the location and severity of a spinal cord or plexus lesion [14]. Birds do not have a cutaneous trunci muscle, and a panniculus reflex cannot be used to help localize a spinal cord lesion; however, the feather follicles contain sensory nerve fibers [65,66]. Tweaking or plucking distinct feathers may be used to determine the level at which touch or pain perception is lost. Light pinpricks lateral to the vertebral column also may assist in localizing a spinal cord lesion. Dermatomes of birds have not been established.

Evaluation of nociception is reserved for those animals showing evidence of spinal cord disease based on abnormalities in proprioception and spinal reflexes. Nociceptive pathways traveling from limb to brain are located deep within the spinal cord. Nociception requires cerebral perception of painful or injurious stimuli. Stimulation begins caudally with a light touch and progresses to deep palpation, a sharp pin prick, and finally a hard pinch. Conscious perception of the pinch stimulus is important in assessing integrity of the spinal cord cranial to the tested limb. Birds may show conscious perception by vocalizing, attempting to bite or escape, or turning to look at the origin of the pain. It is crucial to remember that a withdrawal reflex may be elicited in an animal with a spinal cord that has been transected cranial to the segment responsible for that reflex arc [14,15].

Localization

Disorders should be localized first to a primary division of the nervous system (brain, spinal cord, PNS) and then to its major subdivisions. Table 2 summarizes localization. Injury to the nervous system may cause temporary disturbance or irreversible deficits in function (loss or excess). Abnormalities

Table 2
Localization of neurologic lesions to subdivision of the nervous system in birds according to clinical signs

Region	Local cranial nerve (CN) deficits	Possible clinical signs	
Cerebral cortex	Ipsilateral CN I	Dementia, delirium, seizures	
		Poorly-tuned movement	
		Contralateral proprioceptive loss	
		General/contralateral postural reaction deficits	
		Contralateral vision loss	
Hypothalamus	Ipsilateral CN II	Endocrinopathies	
Rostral brain stem	Ipsilateral CN III-IV	Sleepiness	
-Midbrain		Decerebrate rigidity	
		General/contralateral paresis	
		Strabismus, mydriasis	
Caudal brain stem	Ipsilateral CN V-XII	Irregular respirations	
-Pons		Ataxia, hemi/tetraparesis	
-Medulla		Postural reaction deficits	
		Dysphagia	
		Altered basic instincts	
Cerebellum		Intention tremor	
		Dysmetria, ataxia	
		Incoordination	
Vestibular	CN VIII	Head tilt	
-Central—brain stem		Nystagmus	
-Peripheral—labyrinth		Imbalance, ataxia	
-Paradoxical—caudal cerebellar peduncle		Rolling, circling	
Spinal cord		Cervical	UMN[a] wing and leg
		Brachial plexus	LMN[b] wing, UMN leg
		Thoracic	Normal wing, UMN leg
		Lumbosacral plexus	Normal wing, LMN leg
Diffuse neuromuscular		Decreased reflexes	
		Decreased sensitivity	
		Paresis in all limbs	

[a] *Abbreviation:* UMN, upper motor neuron: paresis or paralysis motor function, normal to increased muscle tone, normal to decreased spinal reflexes, normal to disuse atrophy of muscle mass.

[b] *Abbreviation:* LMN, lower motor neuron: paresis or paralysis motor function, often reduced muscle tone, decreased to absent spinal reflexes, marked neurogenic atrophy of muscle mass.

From Clippinger TL, Bennett RA, Platt SR. The Avian Neurologic Examination and Ancillary Neurodiagnostic Techniques. J Av Med Surg 1996;10(4):221–47; with permission.

may be related to a specific lesion (primary) or to the biochemical events affecting the area surrounding the lesion (secondary). Clinical signs also may reflect attempts of unaffected structures to compensate for dysfunction. Once an anatomic diagnosis is determined, the clinician must select appropriate diagnostic tests to further characterize the lesion or syndrome, to determine etiology, and to help develop a treatment plan [13,16,67].

Diagnostic plan

A minimum database consisting of complete blood count, serum/plasma biochemical analysis, and cytologic evaluation of choanal and cloacal swabs are used to evaluate the contribution of other body systems to the observed clinical signs and physical abnormalities. Additional screening may be indicated depending on clinical signs. Serologic surveys may detect agent antigen or host antibody production related to infectious diseases [68,69] such as chlamydiosis [70,71], aspergillosis [72], sarcocystis [73–75], Newcastle's disease [76,77], Marek's disease [78,79], equine encephalitis virus [80], West Nile virus [81–89], adenovirus [90], and avian influenza [91–93]. Toxologic screening [94,95] for heavy metals [38,40] (eg, lead [16,41,46–48,50,96–98], zinc [99], mercury [49]) and vitamin/mineral assay [30,53,100,101] may differentiate causes of seizures, ataxia, paresis, or paralysis. Low blood cholinesterase concentrations confirm organophosphate or carbamate pesticide poisoning [43,51,97,102–107]. Clinical pathology, diagnostic imaging, electrodiagnostics, and histopathology [26,27] are tools used to confirm and clarify nervous system disease [16,23].

Survey radiography

After a thorough clinical examination, selective or survey radiography may be indicated to evaluate body systems for their contribution to clinical signs. Because it is inexpensive and noninvasive, survey radiography may be one of the best screening tools to uncover a cause for neurologic disease. Survey radiography should be used to evaluate the skull [108,109], axial skeleton, and spinal column, particularly in cases of trauma. Sedation or general anesthesia facilitates exact positioning to yield the best image of the desired area. Both lateral and ventrodorsal projections should be obtained using high-detail film or settings, with the beam centered over the area of interest.

Cerebrospinal fluid analysis

CSF analysis may confirm structural pathologic changes, determine the general nature of the pathologic process, or reveal a specific cause [110,111]. It is most useful in characterizing degenerative, neoplastic, or inflammatory disorders of the spinal cord or brain.

CSF is collected through the foramen magnum between the cerebellum and the dorsal surface of the medulla oblongata. Penetration into the subarachnoid space [55] or into the fourth ventricle rostral to the central canal of the spinal cord allows collection of CSF. The subarachnoid space in birds is narrow, so that fluid collection from the cerebromedullary cistern is difficult. A proliferative network of blood vessels that participates in cerebrospinal production (choroid plexus) lies paramedian bilaterally in the caudomedial aspect of the fourth ventricle [7,55]. Large venous sinuses lie laterally on the interior surface of the occipital bones of the cranial cavity [12]. The collection site must be approached at midline, or significant hemorrhage may occur. Briefly, after flexing the atlanto–occipital joint at a 30-degree angle in a well-aligned laterally recumbent patient, a 25 to 27 gauge needle with a translucent hub is placed at dorsal midline slightly caudal to the occipital protuberance, directed rostrally at a 45-degree angle to the horizontal axis of the head, and advanced slowly through the skin at 1 mm intervals with very controlled motion. In general, 0.1 to 0.5 mL of fluid may be collected [55]. Because of the inherent risk of the cisternal puncture in small avian patients, CSF in birds has not been performed widely.

Sufficient quantities of CSF for gross and microscopic evaluation are collected. The small sample volume usually obtained precludes extensive analysis, but it should be evaluated immediately for its color and clarity and later for its cellular characteristics. Preparation of the CSF sample by cytospin centrifugation is recommended because of the small volume of fluid generally recovered. If a cytocentrifuge is unavailable, the cells may be concentrated by sedimentation on a slide for evaluation of cell concentration, population, and morphology [110,112,113]. Relative erythrocyte and leukocyte numbers and protein level should be compared with that found in the peripheral blood. Meningitis caused by infectious agents generally induces a moderate increase in cell numbers and increased protein content concentration compared with peripheral blood. Noninflammatory conditions caused by degenerative disease or trauma cause a high protein concentration and a minimally increased cell count. CSF evaluation may reveal the disease etiology directly or may complement findings of the clinical presentation to suggest a diagnosis.

Ancillary imaging

Myelography, although in its infancy in avian neurology, may be used to precisely identify the location of spinal cord compression or swelling, especially whenever surgical intervention is contemplated [114,115]. The major technical problems of myelography in birds are the difficulty in inserting the needle into the narrow cerebromedullary cistern and the lack of flow of contrast to the caudal regions of the spinal canal. An iodinated contrast material is injected into the subarachnoid space to provide columns of contrast outlining the course of the spinal cord. A dose of 0.3 mL/kg iohexol (Omnipaque 240) has been recommended and used by the authors with variable results [111].

Myelograms were acquired consistently in 11 normal male pigeons in a recently reported study using the previously described atlanto–occipital space for insertion [115]. A 26 gauge 2.5 cm needle was used to deliver 0.2 mL iohexol over 1 minute. After the head of the subject was elevated for 5 minutes, radiographs were obtained and showed an uninterrupted uniform column extending from the first cervical vertebra to the midcervical region.

The dorsal column was thinner than the ventral column in the caudal cervical region, while both columns were of similar thickness in the cranial cervical region. All birds recovered, and no adverse effects occurred [115].

The fused vertebrae of the synsacrum, the glycogen body, and the absence of a cauda equina interfere with the typical mammalian technique of lumbosacral puncture for subarachnoid access. Using a thoracolumbar approach, a postmortem myelogram was performed in a Red-tailed hawk with paraparesis and demonstrated extravasation of contrast medium in the region of a spinal fracture [114]. In a pilot study of six chickens placed into ventral recumbency in a V-shaped restraint trough, the thoracolumbar site was located by palpation of the first indentation cranial to the synsacrum with the index finger while grasping the thumb and middle finger on the bony prominences of the ileal crests. Survey radiographs, a leg withdrawal reflex upon stimulation of the spinal cord, and the presence of fluid in the hub confirmed proper placement of a 25 gauge, 4 cm spinal needle at the site. Injection of 0.8 to 1.2 mL/kg iohexol contrast medium into the subarachnoid space at 0.5 mL intervals and radiograph acquisition within 10 minutes achieved diagnostic myelograms in four chickens. One subject did not recover after injection of contrast medium into the central canal of the spinal cord. Another subject had right torticollis and paresis after injection of 1.4 mL/kg contrast medium into the appropriate location and evidence of myelogram-induced trauma to the spinal cord on necropsy evaluation 1 week after the myelogram [114].

Nuclear imaging, including brain and bone scintigraphy, may be used as a screening tool in cases of trauma or suspected osteomyelitis whenever survey radiography fails to reveal a lesion [116,117]. A nuclear bone scan may identify metastatic bone lesions, early occult orthopedic injury, avascular necrosis, osteomyelitis, osteoarthritis, and other processes that affect bone turnover. Nuclear bone scanning is particularly useful in identifying spinal abnormalities in birds. In a study involving 12 birds with thoracic or pelvic limb paresis, bone scanning identified 100% of the lesions identified on survey radiographs [118]. In addition, several lesions not identified on survey radiographs, including fractures and early osteomyelitis, were identified by nuclear bone scanning. These pathologic lesions were confirmed by the results of postmortem examination. Brachial vein administration of the radionuclide was found to be superior to medial metatarsal vein administration, possibly because the renal portal system provided high uptake of radionuclide by the liver and kidney and obscured visualization of the spine after medial metatarsal vein administration [118].

CT [119], which uses radiographs and computer technology to create cross-sectional images of the patient [117,120–122], should be used to examine calcified structures [117] or to image soft tissues whenever MRI is unavailable or unmanageable because of anesthetic machine constraints. CT provides superior soft tissue imaging with no superimposition of structures compared with conventional radiography [7,63,117,122,123]. Cross-sectional images may be created at varying intervals with a continuous or noncontinuous technique. Slices most commonly are created every 2 to 3 mm in birds. CT can be used to locate intracranial lesions [124,125]. Acute hematomas are visualized best on CT compared with MRI during the first 24 hours days following traumatic injury. With contrast administration, soft tissues structures are visualized better, especially where there is increased blood flow [125–127]. A dose of 2.22 mg/kg of intravenous iodinated contrast material is recommended. Contrast administration always is recommended to enhance sensitivity, and the degree of contrast enhancement characterizes the degree of blood–brain barrier disruption.

CT has been used to evaluate structures of the avian head [108,120,128] for normality and disease. Multiple imaging modalities were employed to characterize malformations in skull and brain anatomy in the crested breed of the domestic duck (*Anas platyrhynchos* f. dom) [129,130]. Abnormal fatty tissue deposits in the tentorium cerebelli, cranial malformations, and variable bone formations in the thickened hypodermis of the crest were noted on CT [130]. A dorsal laminectomy and spinal stabilization were performed in a traumatically injured umbrella cockatoo (*Cacatua alba*) after survey radiography and CT showed a fractured vertebral body [131]. CT was used to evaluate CNS abnormalities in 10 avian patients in one report [125]. Lesions were identified in 8 of the 10 birds; however, in two birds, no lesions were identified on CT, but histologic lesions were present on postmortem examination. A postmortem CT scan was used to identify spinal cord compression in a juvenile penguin (*Aptenodytes patagonica*) that was euthanized because of an inability to stand despite 6 weeks of medical therapy [132]. Radiographs taken at presentation had failed to identify any spinal abnormalities. Postmortem examination confirmed intervertebral disc rupture and vertebral body displacement.

MRI [117,133] provides excellent soft tissue contrast of the CNS and spatial orientation of anatomic structures. Magnetic resonance imaging (MRI) should be used to evaluate brain and spinal cord soft tissue abnormalities, particularly suspected tumors [122,133,134]. Magnetic resonance imaging has also been employed to evaluate structures of the avian head for normality and disease [135,136].

A high incidence of intracranial tissue deposits, as well as encephaloceles were identified by MRI in domestic ducks (*Anas platyrhynchos* f. dom) with feather crests, a breed with high pre-and postnatal mortality and CNS deficiencies [129]. In a study of normal MRI anatomy of pigeons, imaging required approximately 20 minutes and transverse images were created every 3 mm [137]. Lesions may be missed because of this distance between slices. A continuous technique may be selected to help ameliorate this problem. Decreasing slice thickness to 2 mm decreases image quality but may help to detect small lesions. This imaging modality was used in a clinical case in an attempt to identify the cause of seizure activity in a mealy Amazon parrot (*Amazona farinosa*) [138]. Without contrast enhancement, the lesions were not visualized; however, following the use of contrast material, peri-vascular infiltrates were identified, showing disruption of the blood–brain barrier suggestive of a viral cause.

Electrophysiologic testing

An understanding of myoneuronal electrical activity is essential to interpret an electrodiagnostic evaluation. In the resting state, the inside of a nerve or muscle cell has a net negative electrical potential in relation to the outside of the cell. This difference in charge, the resting potential, is maintained by a series of channels and pumps that transport sodium and potassium ions into and out of the cell. Electrical events, termed action potentials, can be detected only when nerve cells become active or conduct an impulse. Depolarization and action potentials represent the inside of the cell becoming transiently electrically positive with respect to the outside [139].

Electrophysiologic testing is a noninvasive technique used to evaluate the neuromuscular motor unit, which considers the health status of the brain, subcortical nuclei, brainstem nuclei, auditory, visual, olfactory, and sensory areas of the cerebral cortex, and motor and sensory peripheral nerves [16,140–143]. Skeletal and smooth muscle and the myoneural junction may be examined. The muscle and brain are the only areas where continuous activity is evaluated by electromyography (EMG) and electroencephalography (EEG), respectively. Electrical stimulation evokes a response in studies of nerve conduction velocity (NCV).

The device used in clinical neurologic practice to detect these electrical changes is a computer-based system interfaced with differential amplifiers, filters, stimulator, and a signal averaging system (eg, Sapphire 2 ME; TECA Corporation, Pleasantville, New York). The signal averager reduces random artifact by the square root of the number of averages. The quality of the recording also can be improved through selective filtering [143]. Concentric needle electrodes are used to record both the spontaneous and evoked electrical activity of muscle fibers in a small area. Electrodes are usually 27 gauge insulated needles with bare tips that can be inserted into the muscle. A ground electrode must be used always.

Electromyography, nerve conduction studies, and muscle biopsy are used to help differentiate transmission disorder, neuropathy, and myopathy in neuromuscular disease [134,141,143,144]. Motor unit disease may affect any or all components of the motor unit: the ventral horn cell, the spinal root, the nerve root, the peripheral nerve, the neuromuscular junction, or muscle fibers innervated by that nerve. Neuromuscular disease may occur from abnormalities in transmission [145] or from denervation associated with neuropathy or myopathy [146]. Abnormalities in neuromuscular transmission are characterized by generalized weakness and exercise intolerance because of a compromise in patient ability to generate an end plate potential of sufficient amplitude to propagate a muscle action potential [145]. Some insecticides bind acetylcholinesterase, inhibiting neuromuscular transmission. In avian patients, the most common neuromuscular transmission disorder is botulism [39,147–150].

Electromyography

EMG examines the health of the muscle cell and the integrity of the motor unit, consisting of the lower motor neuron (ventral horn cell and motor axon) and the muscle fibers that it innervates. EMG studies the electrical activity of muscle initiated by inserting an electrode into the muscle and recording the electrical activity [142,151]. It is used to confirm a clinical observation of peripheral nerve or muscle disease and may contribute prognostic information [146]. General anesthesia is required for EMG in birds and precludes the use of volitional activity (associated with voluntary muscle contractions) for diagnostic purposes.

Normal resting muscle does not show observable electrical activity with the exception of end-plate noise (spontaneous) associated with resting muscle (Fig. 3). A brief burst of electrical activity (insertional) occurs with needle placement; after stabilization, no audible signal is created [12,131,151]. End-plate potentials (low amplitude [3 to 60 µV] negative discharges) are caused by intermittent release of small amounts of acetylcholine at the neuromuscular junction and are recorded whenever the recording electrode is placed within the end-plate region [152].

A prolonged discharge of insertional potentials sometimes is considered abnormal as it represents cellular irritability. Prolonged insertional activity indicates injury to any portion of the motor unit and does not distinguish neuropathy from myopathy. In dogs and cats, abnormal insertional potentials become noticeable on the fourth or fifth day after muscle denervation and peak in intensity 8 to 10 days after denervation [152]. Potential amplitude, duration, and frequency may be decreased in atrophied muscle [141].

After denervation of muscle, spontaneous, randomly occurring potentials can be demonstrated [152]. These spontaneous potentials, termed fibrillation potentials, are the action potentials of several muscle fibers occurring because of instability in the cell membrane. Time of onset in birds has not been documented, but this may be less than that seen in dogs (5 to 7 days), because earlier onset and greater intensity generally occur in smaller animals [152]. The presence of reproducible discharges in at least two different areas of a single muscle suggests lower motor neuron disease. Fibrillation potentials may indicate a pathologic process involving the ventral horn cell, the nerve root (radiculopathy), the plexus (plexopathy), or axon (mononeuropathy or polyneuropathy) [151]. Muscular pathology occasionally shows low numbers of fibrillation potentials. Fibrillation potentials may not be present if demyelination occurs as a component of a peripheral neuropathy [143]; positive sharp waves (spontaneous electrical potentials that

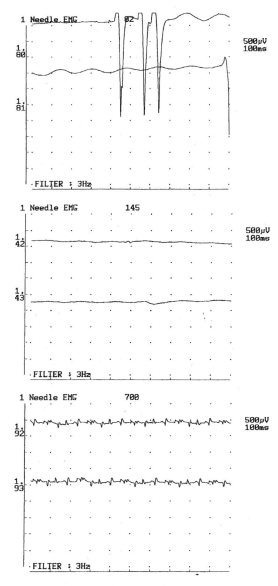

Fig. 3. Electromyograms (EMGs) of a pigeon (*Columba livia*). (*A*) (*top*) Normal insertion potentials recorded as the bipolar electrode is inserted into a muscle. (*B*) (*middle*) Normal muscle is
electrically silent after the bipolar electrode is stabilized. (*C*) (*bottom*) Fibrillation potentials recorded from the pectoral muscle of a pigeon. (*From* Clippinger TL, Bennett RA, Platt SR. The
avian neurologic examination and ancillary neurodiagnostic techniques. J Av Med Surg
1996;10(4):221–47; with permission.)

have a saw tooth appearance) indicate motor unit disorder or muscle disease, and their occurrence may precede fibrillation potentials by one or more days [143]. Fibrillation potentials and occasional bizarre high-frequency discharges suggesting denervation were seen in the wing muscles of red-tailed hawks (*Buteo jamaicensis*) with traumatic brachial plexus injury [153]. Motor unit action potentials observed in these birds suggested that intact nerve fibers were present. With brachial plexus avulsion, a bird is unable to flex its elbow joint, rendering it unable to fly or to hold its wing in a normal folded position. Widespread fibrillation potentials and lack of typical interference potentials supported denervation in the atrophied and/or paretic limbs of three wild birds in another report [154].

Representing a group of muscle fibers firing in near synchrony, complex repetitive discharges are bizarre, high-frequency discharges occurring as rapid, spontaneous, polyphasic potentials. These discharges typically begin suddenly and maintain a constant firing rate, ceasing abruptly and sounding like a machine gun [151]. Complex repetitive discharges may occur in various myopathic conditions including hyperadrenocorticism and polymyositis [143].

Needle EMG has been used to monitor progression and improvement of organophosphate-induced delayed neuropathy in birds [155–162] and zinc-deficiency in chicks [126].

Nerve conduction studies

Nerve conduction studies are a simple and reliable test of peripheral nerve function [151]. Evoked potential amplitude, duration, number of phases, and latency are evaluated. Through electrical stimulation with surface or needle electrodes (cathode and anode) at two sites, an impulse is initiated to travel along a nerve, the M wave (evoked potential) is recorded from a bipolar electrode at the innervated muscle, and a conduction velocity is calculated from the latency of response (Fig. 4). The latency of the response represents the time taken for impulse conduction from the stimulus point along the nerve and the onset of the M wave. Measurement of the distance between the two cathodes that stimulate the nerve at the two different sites is used in an equation to determine the conduction velocity. The conduction velocity is derived from the ratio between the distance (m) described previously and the corresponding latency difference (seconds) of the M waves [151]. Measuring the conduction velocity by two stimulus points on the nerve eliminates time factors required for neuromuscular transmission and generation of a muscle action potential. Separation of the two stimulation points by 10 cm is preferred to improve accuracy, and a 20% to 30% supramaximal intensity is used routinely to guarantee activation of all the nerve axons innervating the recorded muscle [151].

Axonal damage or dysfunction usually will result in loss of amplitude, whereas demyelination leads to prolongation of conduction time (increased

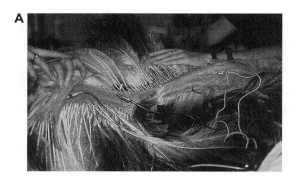

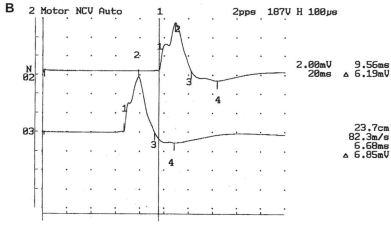

Fig. 4. Nerve conduction velocity study of the ulnar nerve of a rhea (*Rhea americana*). (*A*) (*top*) From left to right, location of the recording bipolar electrode (*gray cable*), ground electrode (*black cable*), and stimulating cathode and anode (*white cables*). (*B*) (*bottom*) Evoked action potential recorded at the ventral interosseous muscle after electrical stimulation of the ulnar nerve.

latency) [151]. Reduced amplitude may occur 48 hours after complete nerve transection [151]. With demonstration of reduced amplitude and normal velocity in the first few days after peripheral nerve injury, neurapraxia (transient loss of function) is difficult to differentiate from early axonotmesis (axon disruption with internal fiber preservation). This distinction can be made by stimulating the nerve distal to the lesion later in the disease course when the degenerating axons have lost their excitability [151]. Increased latency with a normal amplitude indicates segmental demyelination affecting most of the nerve fibers. Increased latency also may result from axonal neuropathy with the loss of fast conducting fibers, but this usually will be accompanied by a 50% reduction in amplitude.

Regardless of the amplitude, a conduction velocity reduced to less than 60% of the mean normal value suggests peripheral nerve disease rather than spinal cord disease [163]. In a severed canine motor nerve, conduction within the distal stump stops abruptly after about 5 to 8 days because of Wallerian degeneration of the distal stump [152]. Absent responses indicate conduction failure in most nerve fibers, implying neurapraxia, axonotmesis, or nerve transection. In any case, it must be kept in mind that nerve stimulation distal to the lesion will elicit a normal muscle action potential for several days after initial injury.

In birds, mean ischiatic nerve conduction velocities have been determined in studies by percutaneous stimulation at the level of the tibial nerve and recording from the digital flexor muscles in various avian species, including white leghorn hens older than 2 years (60 m/s, n = 12 [158]) and adult pigeons (46.56 m/s, n = 26 [164]). Mean values for tibial nerve conduction velocities are available from other experimental studies:

- White leghorn hens older than 2 years (41 m/s, n = 12 [158]),
- 2- to 4-week-old white leghorn chickens (32.3 m/s, n = 65 [165]),
- 15-week-old chickens (53 m/s, n = 53 [166]),
- Adult barred owls (*Strix varia*, 134.2 m/s, n = 6 [167]),
- Adult rheas (*Rhea americana*, 129.8 m/s, n = 6 [167])

Ulnar NCV was derived for rheas (62.9 m/s, n = 6 [167]), barred owls (56.6 m/s n = 6 [167]), and pigeons (52.4 m/s, n = 26 [164]).

Generally, NCVs are faster at higher body temperatures [152,168], in adults that have increased mean fiber diameter compared with developing animals [152,166], and in shorter nerves [151,169]. In chickens, motor NCV increased from approximately 23 m/s at 1 week of age to 53 m/sec at 15 weeks of age [166].

Despite certain limitations, measurement of motor NCV may provide pertinent diagnostic information if interpreted judiciously in appropriate clinical contexts [151].

The F wave

Measurement of the F wave, an evoked muscle response, can help in the assessment of motor conduction along the most proximal segment of a nerve. The F wave arises after the M wave and results from the backfiring of the ventral horn cell located in the spinal cord (Fig. 5). Its measurement, termed the F latency, supplements conventional nerve conduction studies, especially in patients with proximal polyneuropathies where delay of the F wave may exceed the normal range markedly [16,152,170].

Repetitive stimulation

Repeated supramaximal stimulation should create repeatable identical action potentials in normal patients (Fig. 6). Any evidence of an incremental or decremental response may have physiological significance. Any defect in neuromuscular transmission usually will produce a maximal drop in amplitude between the first and second responses of a train, followed by gradual

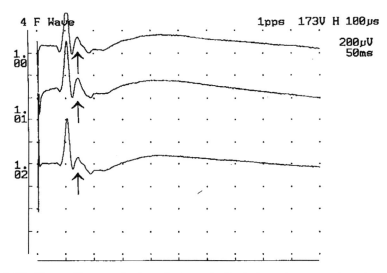

Fig. 5. The F wave. Nerve conduction velocity study. Evoked muscle response (*arrow*) resulting from antidromic propagation of the ischiatic nerve impulse following electrical stimulation in a barred owl (*Strix varia*). The F response occurs following the M wave after supramaximal stimulation.

decline to the fourth or fifth potential, where it levels off [151]. Agents that increase the concentration of acetylcholine at the neuromuscular junction block this decremental tendency. Botulism targets the presynaptic nerve terminal and causes a tendency for an incremental response to repetitive stimulation [131,151,152].

Muscle biopsy

Muscle biopsy is indicated to confirm, define, and possibly provide a cause for motor unit disease [145,171]. Often, the biopsy is obtained immediately from the affected muscle and its opposite muscle following electrophysiologic testing. The muscle selected for biopsy should be one that is affected clinically with the disease process. In acute disease, a severely affected muscle is selected. With chronic disease, a muscle demonstrating only moderate changes is the best choice. The chosen site should allow biopsy of the muscle and associated nerves without affecting other surrounding structures. The incision is made through the skin and muscle fascia to expose the muscle fibers. A portion of the muscle fibers is grasped with forceps, and a cylindrical portion is cut out with sharp microscissors. After collection of two to three samples, closure is routine. The biopsy is placed on and covered with a saline-moistened gauze, refrigerated, and sent for evaluation as soon as possible, as viability markedly decreases within 30 hours. The sample should not be fixed in formalin or stretched. Enzyme histochemical staining is used to determine the distribution of fiber types (I, IIA, IIB).

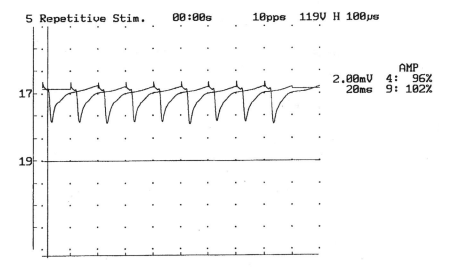

Fig. 6. Repetitive stimulation. Identical action potentials created by supramaximal stimulation (ten pulses per second at 119 V) of the ischiatic nerve and reflecting the similar number of muscle fibers activated by nerve impulses each time in a pigeon (*Columba livia*). Note that the ninth wave is 102% of the first wave, a normal response. (*From* Clippinger TL, Bennett RA, Platt SR. The avian neurologic examination and ancillary neurodiagnostic techniques. J Av Med Surg 1996;10(4):221–47; with permission.)

Typically, muscles chosen for biopsy would be ones for which normal fiber type, distribution, and size are known; however, this information is not available for most avian patients [2]. Parameters usually evaluated include mean muscle fiber diameter, percent fiber types, percent internal nuclei, variability coefficient, and atrophy and hypertrophy factors [171]. In addition to characterizing myopathy secondary to diseases of the motor unit, histopathologic evaluation of muscle may reveal the presence of an infectious disease agent, such as *Sarcocystis* species [27,74,75,172–174].

Electroencephalography

EEG is the study of the electrical events that occur in the cerebral cortex. The electroencephalogram is the permanent record of these events and represents the summation of variable resting potentials of the neurons in the cortex, the excitatory and inhibitory resting postsynaptic potentials, and possibly the action potentials of the cortical neurons (Fig. 7) [175]. Classic studies conducted primarily in chickens showed effects related to various stimuli:

- Photic (slow, high-amplitude waves associated with darkness)
- Acoustic (reduced amplitude associated with sound)
- Anesthetic (spike pattern associated with barbiturates)
- Temperature (decreased amplitude associated with hypothermia) [176]

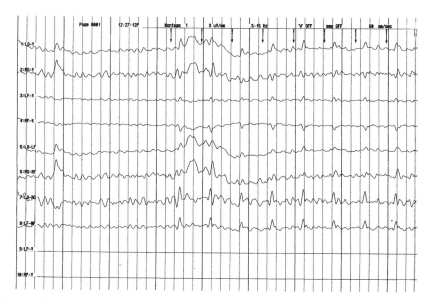

Fig. 7. Electroencephalogram of the avian cortex with an eight-channel montage, recorded from an anesthetized pigeon (*Columba livia*) at rest and following a stroboscopic flash. The negative deflection of the line at the tip of the tracing indicates initiation of the stimulus. (*From* Clippinger TL, Bennett RA, Platt SR. The avian neurologic examination and ancillary neuro-diagnostic techniques. J Av Med Surg 1996;10(4):221–47; with permission.)

Variations of normality and differences across species exist, causing considerable difficulty in interpretating results. In general, interpretation has been associated with patient age and level of consciousness (alert: high-frequency/low-voltage; relaxed: low-frequency/high-voltage; sleep: irregular low-frequency/very high voltage discharges) [139]. Disease may cause changes in either amplitude (most dramatic) or frequency (more reliable) and occasionally in both. Pattern spikes indicate an area of irritability and may be associated with a seizure focus [139]. The electroencephalogram is not a specific test; asymmetry in EEG recordings may aid interpretation.

Summary

Physical and neurologic examinations identify neurologic dysfunction and the corresponding anatomic location of the lesion. Ancillary diagnostic tests confirm and clarify conclusions from the neurologic examination and often identify the cause of disease. CSF analysis, diagnostic imaging, electrodiagnostics, and histopathology are important tools in avian neurology. Further research, evaluation, and experience are necessary to refine use of these tools for the avian practitioner. Once the disease location and pathologic process have been identified, appropriate treatment and prognosis may be provided.

References

[1] Bennett RA. Neurology. In: Ritchie BW, Harrison GJ, Harrison LR, editors. Avian medicine: principles and application. Lake Worth (FL): Wingers Publishing; 1994. p. 728–47.

[2] Benzo CA. Nervous system. In: Sturkie PD, editor. Avian physiology. 4th edition. New York: Springer-Verlag; 1986. p. 1–37.

[3] Dubbeldam JL. Motor control system. In: Sturkie PD, editor. Avian physiology. 5th edition. New York: Springer-Verlag; 2000. p. 83–99.

[4] Evans HE. Anatomy of the budgerigar. In: Petrak ML, editor. Diseases of cage and aviary birds. 2nd edition. Philadelphia: Lea & Febiger; 1982. p. 111–87.

[5] Kern TJ. Disorders of the special senses. In: Altman RB, Clubb SL, Dorrestein GM, et al, editors. Avian medicine and surgery. Philadelphia: WB Saunders Co.; 1997. p. 563–89.

[6] Necker R. Functional organization of the spinal cord. In: Sturkie PD, editor. Avian physiology. 5th edition. New York: Springer-Verlag; 2000. p. 71–81.

[7] Nickel R, Schummer A, Sieferle E, et al. Anatomy of the domestic birds. Berlin: Verlag Paul Parey; 1977.

[8] Orosz SE. Principles of avian clinical neuroanatomy. Sem Av Ex Pet Med 1996;5(3):127–39.

[9] Sturkie PD, Whittow GC, editors. Sturkie's avian physiology. 5th edition. San Diego (CA): Academic Press, Harcourt Brace and Co.; 2000.

[10] Willis AM, Wilkie DA. Avian ophthalmology part 1: anatomy, examination, and diagnostic techniques. J Avian Med Surg 1999;13(3):160–6.

[11] Clippinger TL, Bennett RA, Platt SR. The avian neurologic examination and ancillary neurodiagnostic techniques. J Avian Med Surg 1996;10(4):221–47.

[12] De Lahunta A. Veterinary neuroanatomy and clinical neurology. 2nd edition. Philadelphia: WB Saunders Co.; 1983.

[13] Jones MP, Orosz SE. Overview of avian neurology and neurological diseases. Sem Av Ex Pet Med 1996;5(3):150–64.

[14] Oliver JE, Lorenz MD, Kornegay JN. Handbook of veterinary neurology. 4th edition. Philadelphia: WB Saunders; 2004.

[15] Schunk KL. Neurologic emergencies. In: Murtaugh RJ, Kaplan PM, editors. Veterinary emergency and critical care medicine. St Louis (MO): Mosby-Yearbook Inc; 1992. p. 288–94.

[16] Platt SR. Evaluating and treating the nervous system. In: Harrison GJ, Lightfoot TL, editors. Clinical avian medicine: volume II. Palm Beach (FL): Spix Publishing; 2006. p. 493–517.

[17] Thomas WB. Initial assessment of patients with neurologic dysfunction. Vet Clin North Am Small Anim Pract 2000;30(1):1–24.

[18] Wheeler SJ, editor. Manual of small animal neurology. 2nd edition. Sturdington (UK): British Small Animal Veterinary Association; 1995.

[19] Clippinger TL, Platt SR. Seizures. In: Olsen GH, Orosz SE,, editors. Manual of avian medicine. St Louis (MO): Mosby Inc; 2000. p. 170–82.

[20] Carleton RE, Garner MM, Nayden D. Malignant astrocytoma with characteristics of a glioblastoma multiforme in a green-cheeked conure (*Pyrrhura molinae*). J Avian Med Surg 2004;18(4):106–10.

[21] Dyer SM, Keating J, Ewing PJ, et al. A primitive neuroectodermal tumor in the cerebellum of an umbrella cockatoo (*Cacatua alba*). J Avian Med Surg 2003;17(1):20–6.

[22] Johnston HA, Lindstrom JG, Oglesbee M. Communicating hydrocephalus in a mature Goffin's cockatoo (*Cacatua goffini*). J Avian Med Surg 2006;20(3):180–4.

[23] Larsen RS, Nutter FB, Augspurger T, et al. Clinical features of avian vacuolar myelinopathy in American coots. J Am Vet Med Assoc 2002;221(1):80–5.

[24] Rocke TE, Thomas NJ, Augspurger T, et al. Epizootioligic studies of avian vacuolar myelinopathy in waterbirds. J Wildl Dis 2002;38(4):678–84.

[25] Romagnano A, Mashima TY, Barnes HJ. Pituitary adenoma in an Amazon parrot. J Avian Med Surg 1995;9(4):263–70.

[26] Schmidt RE, Reavill DR, Phalen DN. Pathology of pet and aviary birds. Ames (IA): Iowa State Press; 2003. p. 165–176.

[27] Shivaprasad HL. Disease of the nervous system in pet birds: a review and report of diseases rarely documented. Proc Assoc Avian Vet 1993;213–22.

[28] Suchy A, Weissenbock H, Schmidt P. Intracranial tumors in budgerigars. Avian Pathol 1999;28:125–30.

[29] Berhane Y, Smith DA, Newman S, et al. Peripheral neuritis in psittacine birds with proventricular dilatation disease. Avian Pathol 2001;30:563–70.

[30] Johnston MS, Ivey ES. Parathyroid and ultimobranchial glands: calcium metabolism in birds. Sem Av Exotic Ped Med 2002;11(2):84–93.

[31] Forbes NA, Simpson GN. Caryospora neofalconis: an emerging threat to captive-bred raptors in the United Kingdom. J Avian Med Surg 1997;11(2):110–4.

[32] Hawkins MG, Couto S, Tell LA, et al. Atypical parasitic migration and necrotizing sacral myelitis due to serratospiculoides amaculata in a prairie falcon (Falco mexicanus). Avian Dis 2001;45(1):276–83.

[33] Kirkpatrick CE, Colvin BA, Dubey JP. Toxoplasma gondii antibodies in common barn owls (Tyto alga) and pigeons (Columba livia) in New Jersey. Vet Parasitol 1990;36: 177–80.

[34] Monks DJ, Carlisle MS, Carrigan M, et al. Angiostsrongylus cantonensis as a cause of cerebrospinal disease in a yellow-tailed black cockatoo (Calyptorhynchus funereus) and two tawny frogmouths (Podargus strigoides). J Avian Med Surg 2005;19(4):289–93.

[35] Spalding MG, Yowell CA, Lindsay DS, et al. Sarcocystis meningoencephalitis in a northern gannet (Morus bassanus). J Wildl Dis 2002;38(2):432–7.

[36] Williams CK, McKown RD, Veatch JK, et al. Baylisascaris sp found in a wild northern bobwhite (Colinus virginianus). J Wildl Dis 1997;33(1):158–60.

[37] Williams SM, Fulton RM, Render JA, et al. Ocular and encephalic toxoplasmosis in canaries. Avian Dis 2001;45(1):262–7.

[38] Bauck L, LaBonde J. Toxic disorders. In: Altman RB, Clubb SL, Dorrestein GM, editors. Avian medicine and surgery. Philadelphia: WB Saunders Co.; 1997. p. 604–13.

[39] Campbell TW. Crown vetch (Coronilla varia) poisoning in a budgerigar (Melopsittacus undulatus). J Avian Med Surg 2006;20(2):97–100.

[40] Dumonceaux G, Harrison GJ. Toxins. In: Ritchie BW, Harrison GJ, Harrison LR, editors. Avian medicine: principles and application. Lake Worth (FL): Wingers Publishing; 1994. p. 1030–52.

[41] Kramer L, Redig PT. Sixteen years of lead poisoning in eagles, 1980–95: an epizootiologic view. J Raptor Res 1997;31:327–32.

[42] Kreuder C, Mazet JAK, Bossart GD, et al. Clinicopathologic features of suspected brevetoxicosis in double-crested cormorants (Phalacrocorax auritus) along the Florida gulf coast. J Zoo Wildl Med 2002;33(1):8–15.

[43] LaBonde J. Toxicity in pet avian patients. Sem Avian Exotic Pet Med 1995;4:23–31.

[44] LaBonde J. Two clinical cases of exposure to household use of organophosphate and carbamate insecticides. Proc Assoc Avian Vet 1992;113–8.

[45] Lewis LA, Schweitzer SH. Lead poisoning in a northern bobwhite in Georgia. J Wildl Dis 2000;36(1):150–3.

[46] Mateo R, Carles-Dolz J, Aguilar JM, et al. An epizootic of lead poisoning in greater flamingos (Phoenicoperus ruber roseus) in Spain. J Wildl Dis 1997;33(1):135–9.

[47] Mautino M. Lead and zinc intoxication in zoological medicine: a review. J Zoo Wildl Med 1997;28(1):28–35.

[48] Shimmel L, Snell K. Case studies in poisoning: two eagles. Sem Av Exotic Pet Med 1999; 8(1):12–20.

[49] Spalding MG, Frederick PC, McGill HC, et al. Histologic, neurologic, and immunologic effects of methylmercury in captive great egrets. J Wildl Dis 2000;36(3):423–35.

[50] Wilson HM, Oyen JL, Sileo L. Lead shot poisoning of a Pacific loon in Alaska. J Wildl Dis 2004;40(3):600–2.

[51] Wobeser G, Bollinger T, Leighton FA, et al. Secondary poisoning of eagles following intentional poisoning of coyotes with anticholinesterase pesticides in Western Canada. J Wildl Dis 2004;40(2):163–72.

[52] Holz PH, Phelan JR, Slocombe R. Thiamine deficiency in honeyeaters. J Avian Med Surg 2002;16(1):21–5.

[53] Smith JM, Roudybus TE. Nutritional disorders. In: Altman RB, Clubb SL, Dorrestein GM, et al, editors. Avian medicine and surgery. Philadelphia: WB Saunders Co.; 1997. p. 501–16.

[54] Bolton TB. The structure of the nervous system & the physiology of the nervous system. In: Bell DJ, Freeman GM, editors. Physiology and biochemistry of the domestic fowl. London: Academic Press; 1971. p. 641–73, 675–705.

[55] King AS, McClelland J. Birds-their structure and function. 2nd edition. London: Bailliére Tindall; 1984. p. 237–315.

[56] Rosenthal K, Orosz S, Dorrestein GM. Nervous system. In: Altman RB, Clubb SL, Dorrestein GM, et al, editors. Avian medicine and surgery. Philadelphia: WB Saunders Co.; 1997. p. 454–74.

[57] Li T, Howland HC. A true neuronal consensual pupillary reflex in chicks. Vision Res 1999; 39(5):897–900.

[58] Bravo H, Inzunza O. The oculomotor nucleus, not the abducent, innervates the muscles which advance the nictitating membrane in birds. Acta Anat 1985;122:99–104.

[59] Gancz AY, Malka S, Sandmeyer L, et al. Horner's syndrome in a red-bellied parrot (Poicephalus rufiventris). J Avian Med Surg 2005;19(1):30–4.

[60] Williams DL, Cooper JE. Horner's syndrome in an African spotted eagle owl (Bubo africanus). Vet Rec 1994;134:64–6.

[61] Malka S, Keirstead ND, Gancz AY, et al. Ingluvial squamous cell carcinoma in a geriatric cockatiel (Nymphicus hollandicus). J Avian Med Surg 2005;19(3):234–9.

[62] Sanchez C, Bush M, Montali R. Polycystic kidney disease associated with unilateral lameness in a Northern pintail (Anas acuta). J Avian Med Surg 2004;18(4):257–62.

[63] Orosz SE, Ensley PK, Haynes CJ. Avian surgical anatomy-thoracic and pelvic limbs. Philadelphia: WB Saunders; 1992.

[64] Fowler ME. Clinical anatomy of ratites. In: Fowler ME, editor. Zoo and wild animal medicine-current therapy 3. Philadelphia: WB Saunders; 1993. p. 194–8.

[65] Bauck L, Orosz S, Dorrestein GM. Avian dermatology. In: Altman RB, Clubb SL, Dorrestein GM, editors. Avian medicine and surgery. Philadelphia: WB Saunders Co.; 1997. p. 540–62.

[66] Cooper JE, Harrison GJ. Dermatology. In: Ritchie BW, Harrison GJ, Harrison LR, editors. Avian medicine: principles and application. Lake Worth (FL): Wingers Publishing; 1994. p. 607–39.

[67] Platt SR, Clippinger TL. Neurologic Signs. In: Olsen GH, Orosz SE, editors. Manual of avian medicine. St Louis (MO): Mosby Inc; 2000. p. 148–69.

[68] Phalen D. Implications of viruses in clinical disorders. In: Harrison GJ, Lightfoot TL, editors. Clinical avian medicine: volume II. Palm Beach (FL): Spix Publishing; 2006. p. 721–45.

[69] Phalen D. The use of serologic assays in avian medicine. Sem Av Exotic Pet Med 2001;10(2): 77–89.

[70] Flammer K. Chlamydiosis. In: Fowler ME, Miller ER, editors. Zoo & wildlife medicine. 5th edition. Philadelphia: Saunders, Elsevier Science; 2003. p. 718–23.

[71] Tully TN. Update on Chlamydophila psittaci. Sem Av Exotic Pet Med 2001;10(1):20–4.

[72] Redig PT. Aspergillosis. In: Samour J, editor. Avian medicine. Philadelphia: Mosby; 2000. p. 275–87.
[73] Cray C, Zielenzienski-Roberts K, Bonda M, et al. Serologic diagnosis of sarcocystis in psittacine birds: 16 birds. J Avian Med Surg 2005;19(3):208–15.
[74] Dubey JR, Johnson GC, Bermudez A, et al. Neural sarcocystosis in a straw-necked ibis (*Carphibis spinicollis*) associated with a *Sarcocystis neurona*-like organism and description of muscular sarcocysts of an unidentified *Sarcocystis* species. J Parasitol 2001;87(6): 1317–22.
[75] Siegal-Willot JL, Pollock CG, Carpenter JW, et al. Encephalitis caused by *Sarcocystis falcatula*-like organisms in a white cockatoo (*Cacatua alba*). J Avian Med Surg 2005; 19(1):19–24.
[76] Kuiken T, Leighton FA, Wobeser G, et al. An epidemic of Newcastle disease in double-crested cormorants from Saskatchewan. J Wildl Dis 1998;34:457–71.
[77] Kuiken T, Wobeser G, Leighton FA, et al. Pathology of Newcastle disease in double-crested cormorants from Saskatchewan, with comparison of diagnostic methods. J Wildl Dis 1999;35(1):8–23.
[78] Gimeno IM, Witter RL, Reed WM. Four distinct neurologic syndromes in Marek's disease: effect of viral strain and pathotype. Avian Dis 1999;43(4):721–37.
[79] Terrell SP, Romero CH, Schutzi PJ. The pathology associated with an outbreak of Marek's disease in green junglefowl (*Gallus varius*). Proc Am Assoc Zoo Vet 2004;447–8.
[80] Tuttle AD, Andreadis TG, Frasca S, et al. Eastern equine encephalitis in a flock of African penguins maintained at an aquarium. J Am Vet Med Assoc 2005;226(12):2059–62.
[81] Bertelsen MF, Ølberg RA, Crawshaw GJ, et al. West Nile virus infection in the Eastern loggerhead shrike (*Lanius ludovicianus migrans*): pathology, epidemiology, and immunization. J Wildl Dis 2004;40(3):538–42.
[82] D'Agostino JJ, Isaza R. Clinical signs and results of specific diagnostic testing among captive birds housed at zoological institutions and infected with West Nile virus. J Am Vet Med Assoc 2004;224(10):1640–3.
[83] Fitzgerald SD, Patterson JS, Kiupel M, et al. Clinical and pathologic features of West Nile virus infection in native North American owls (Family strigidae). Avian Dis 2003;47(3): 602–10.
[84] Kramer LD, Bernard KA. West Nile infection in birds and mammals. Ann N Y Acad Sci 2001;951:84–93.
[85] Ludwig GV, Calle PP, Mangiafico JA, et al. An outbreak of West Nile virus in a New York City captive wildlife population. Am J Trop Med Hyg 2002;67(1):67–75.
[86] Wunschmann A, Shivers J, Bender J, et al. Pathologic findings in red-tailed hawks (*Buteo jamaicensis*) and Cooper's hawks (*Accipiter cooper*) naturally infected with West Nile virus. Avian Dis 2004;48(3):570–80.
[87] Roehrig Jt, Layton M, Smith P, et al. The emergence of West Nile virus in North America: ecology, epidemiology, and surveillance. Curr Top Microbiol Immunol 2002;267:223–40.
[88] Steele KE, Linn MJ, Schoepp RJ, et al. Pathology of fatal West Nile virus infections in native and exotic birds during the 1999 outbreak in New York City, New York. Vet Pathol 2000;37:208–24.
[89] Wunschmann A, Shivers J, Bender J, et al. Pathologic and immunohistochemical findings in goshawks (*Accipiter gentilis*) and great horned owls (*Bubo virginianus*) naturally infected with West Nile virus. Avian Dis 2005;49(2):252–9.
[90] Zsivanovits P, Monks DJ, Forbes NA, et al. Presumptive identification of a novel adenovirus in a Harris hawk (*Parabuteo unicinctus*), a Bengal eagle owl (*Bubo bengalensis*), and a Verreaux's eagle owl (*Bubo lacteus*). J Avian Med Surg 2006;20(2):105–12.
[91] Perkins LE, Swayne DE. Pathobiology of A/chicken/HongKong/220/97 (H5N1) avian influenza virus in seven *Gallinaceous* species. Vet Pathol 2001;38:149–64.
[92] Perkins LE, Swayne DE. Pathogenicity of a Hong Kong-origin H5N1 highly pathogenic avian influenza virus for emus, geese, ducks, and pigeons. Avian Dis 2002;46(1):53–63.

[93] Perkins LE, Swayne DE. Varied pathogenicity of a Hong Kong-origin H5N1 avian influenza virus in four passerine species and budgerigars. Vet Pathol 2003;40(1):14–24.

[94] Degernes LA. Toxicities in waterfowl. Sem Avian Exotic Pet Med 1995;4:15–22.

[95] Woods LW, Plumlee KH. Avian toxicoses: veterinary diagnostic laboratory perspective. Sem Av Exotic Pet Med 1999;8(1):32–5.

[96] Brown CS, Luebbert J, Mulcahy D, et al. Rosenberg. Blood lead levels of wild Steller's eiders (*Polysticita stelleri*) and black scoters (*Melanitta nigra*) in Alaska using a portable blood lead analyzer. J Zoo Wildl Med 2006;37(3):361–5.

[97] Franson JC, Smith MR. Poisoning of wild birds from exposure to anticholinesterase compounds and lead: diagnostic methods and selected cases. Sem Av Exotic Pet Med 1999;8(1):3–11.

[98] Samour JH, Naldo J. Diagnosis and therapeutic management of lead toxicosis in falcons in Saudi Arabia. J Avian Med Surg 2002;16(1):16–20.

[99] Holz PH. Suspected zinc toxicosis as a cause of sudden death in orange-bellied parrots (*Neophema chrysogaster*). J Avian Med Surg 2000;14(1):37–41.

[100] Aye PP, Morishita TY, Grimes S, et al. Encephalomalacia associated with vitamin E deficiency in commercially raised emus. Avian Dis 1998;42(3):600–5.

[101] Torregrossa AM, Puschner B, Tell LA, et al. Circulating concentrations of vitamins A and E in captive psittacine birds. J Avian Med Surg 2005;19(3):225–9.

[102] Burn JD, Leighton FA. Further studies of brain cholinesterase: cholinergic receptor ratios in the diagnosis of acute lethal poisoning of birds by anticholinesterase pesticides. J Wildl Dis 1996;32(2):216–24.

[103] Elliott JE, Langelier KM, Mineaus P, et al. Poisoning of bald eagles and red-tailed hawks by carbofuran and fensulfothian in the Fraser Delta of British Columbia, Canada. J Wildl Dis 1996;32(3):486–91.

[104] Garcelon DK, Thomas NJ. DDE poisoning in an adult bald eagle. J Wildl Dis 1997;33(2):299–303.

[105] Hunt KA, Hooper Mj, Edward EL. Carbofuran poisoning in herons: cholinesterase reactivation techniques. J Wildl Dis 1995;31(2):186–92.

[106] Small MF, Pruett CL, Hewitt DG, et al. Cholinseterase activity in white-winged doves exposed to methyl parathion. J Wildl Dis 1998;34(4):698–703.

[107] Tully TN, Osofsky A, Jowett PLH, et al. Acetylcholinesterase concentrations in heparinized blood of Hispaniolan Amazon parrots (*Amazona ventralis*). J Zoo Wildl Med 2003;34(4):411–3.

[108] Krautwald-Junghanns ME, Pees M. Radiographic diagnosis of the head. Proc Assoc Av Vet 2005;51–6.

[109] Paul-Murphy JR, Koblik PD, Stein G, et al. Psittacine skull radiography: anatomy, radiographic technic, and patient application. Vet Radiol 1990;31(4):218–24.

[110] Chrisman CL. Cerebrospinal fluid analysis. Vet Clin North Am Small Anim Pract 1992;22(4):781–810.

[111] Klappenbach KM. Cerebral spinal fluid analysis in psittacines. Proc Assoc Avian Vet 1995;39–42.

[112] Campbell TW. Avian hematology and cytology. Ames (IA): Iowa State University Press; 1992. p. 33–40.

[113] Campbell TW. Concentrating fluids for cytologic exam. J Assoc Avian Vet 1992;6(2):92.

[114] Harr KE, Kollias GV, Rendano V, et al. A myelographic technique for avian species. Vet Radiol Ultrasound 1997;38(3):187–92.

[115] Nacini AT, Dadras H, Naeini BA. Myelography in the pigeon (*Columba livia*). J Avian Med Surg 2006;20(1):27–30.

[116] Brawner WR, Daniel GB. Nuclear imaging. Vet Clin North Am Small Anim Pract 1993;23(2):379–98.

[117] Stoskopf MK. Clinical imaging in zoological medicine: a review. J Zoo Wildl Med 1989;20(4):396–412.

[118] Lung NP, Ackerman N. Scintigraphy as a tool in avian orthopedic diagnosis. Proc Am Assoc Zoo Vet 1993;45.

[119] Berry CR. Physical principles of computed tomography and magnetic resonance imaging. In: Thrall DE, editor. Textbook of veterinary diagnostic radiology. 4th edition. Philadelphia: WB Saunders Co; 2002. p. 28–35.

[120] Krautwald-Junghanns ME, Kostka VM, Dörsch B. Comparative studies on the diagnostic value of conventional radiography and computed tomography in evaluating the heads of psittacine and raptorial birds. J Avian Med Surg 1998;12(3):149–57.

[121] Krautwald-Junghanns ME, Tellhelm B. Advances in radiography of birds. Sem Avian Exotic Pet Med 1994;3(3):115–25.

[122] Sande RD. Radiography, myelography, computed tomography, and magnetic resonance imaging of the spine. Vet Clin North Am Small Anim Pract 1992;22(4):811–31.

[123] Love N, Flammer K, Spaulding K. The normal computed tomographic (CT) anatomy of the African grey parrot (Psittacus erithacus): a pilot study. Proc Amer Coll Vet Radiol 1993;28.

[124] Jenkins JR. Use of computed tomography (CT) in pet bird practice. Proc Assoc Avian Vet 1991;276–9.

[125] Rosenthal K, Stefanacci J, Quesenberry K, et al. Computerized tomography in 10 cases of avian intracranial disease. Proc Assoc Avian Vet 1995;305.

[126] O'Dell BL, Conley-Harrison J, Browning JD, et al. Zinc deficiency and peripheral neuropathy in chicks. Proc Soc Exp Biol Med 1990;194(1):1–4.

[127] Orosz SE, Toal RL. Tomographic anatomy of the golden eagle (Aquila chrysaetos). J Zoo Wildl Med 1992;23(1):39–46.

[128] Gumpenberger M, Kolm G. Ultrasongraphic and computed tomographic examinations of the avian eye: physiologic appearnce, pathologic findings, and comparative biometric measurement. Vet Radiol Ultrasound 2006;47(5):492–502.

[129] Bartels T, Brinkmeier J, Portmann S, et al. Magnetic resonance imaging of intracranial tissue accumulations in domestic ducks (Anas platyrhynchos f. dom) with feather crests. Vet Radiol Ultrasound 2001;42(3):254–8.

[130] Bartels T, Krautwald-Junghanns M-E, Portmann S, et al. The use of conventional radiography and computer-assisted tomography as instruments for demonstration of gross pathological lesions in the cranium and cerebrum in the crested breed of the domestic duck (Anas platyrhynchos f. dom.). Avian Pathol 2000;29:101–8.

[131] Powers LV, Bergman RL. Surgical spinal stabilization in an umbrella cockatoo (Cacatua alba). Proc Assoc Avian Vet 2005;341–7.

[132] Emerson CL, Eurell JC, Brown MD, et al. Ruptured intervertebral disc in a juvenile king penguin (Aptenodytes patagonica). J Zoo Wildl Med 1990;21(3):345–50.

[133] Thomson CE, Kornegay JN, Burn RA, et al. Magnetic resonance imaging—a general overview of principles and examples in veterinary neurodiagnosis. Vet Radiol Ultrasound 1993; 34(1):2–17.

[134] Coates JR. Intervertebral disk disease. Vet Clin North Am Small Anim Pract 2000;30(1): 77–110.

[135] Morgan RV, Donnell RL, Daniel GB. Magnetic resonance imaging of the normal eye and orbit of a screech owl (Otus asio). Vet Radiol Ultrasound 1994;35(5):362–7.

[136] Pye GW, Bennett RA, Newell SM, et al. Magnetic resonance imaging in psittacine birds with chronic sinusitis. J Avian Med Surg 2000;14(4):243–56.

[137] Romagnano A. Magnetic resonance imaging of the brain and coelomic cavity of the domestic pigeon (Columba livia domestica). Vet Radiol Ultrasound 1996;37(6):431–40.

[138] Romagnano A, Shiroma JT, Heard DJ, et al. Magnetic resonance imaging of the avian brain and abdominal cavity. Proc Assoc Avian Vet 1995;307–9.

[139] Redding RW. Electroencephalography. Prog Vet Neuro 1990;1(2):181–7.

[140] Hendrix DV, Sims MH. Electroretinography in the Hispaniolan Amazon parrot (Amazona ventralis). J Avian Med Surg 2004;18(2):89–94.

[141] Klappenbach KM. Neuroelectrodiagnostics in psittacines. Proc Assoc Avian Vet 1995;37–8.
[142] Lipsitz D. Electromyography and nerve conduction velocity studies. In: Ettinger SJ, Feldman EC, editors. Textbook of veterinary internal medicine. 6th edition. St Louis (MO): Elsevier Inc; 2005. p. 328–9.
[143] Sims MH. Clinical electrodiagnostic evaluation in exotic animal medicine. Sem Av Ex Pet Med 1996;5(3):140–9.
[144] Glass EN, Kent M. The clinical examination for neuromuscular disease. Vet Clin North Am Small Anim Pract 2002;32(1):1–31.
[145] Shelton GD. Disorders of neuromuscular transmission. Semin Vet Med Surg 1989;4(2): 126–32.
[146] Platt SR. Peripheral neuropathy in a turkey vulture with lead toxicosis. J Am Vet Med Assoc 1999;214(8):1218–20.
[147] Cambre RC. Water quality for a waterfowl collection. In: Fowler ME, Miller ER, editors. Zoo & wildlife medicine: current therapy 4. Philadelphia: WB Saunders Co.; 1999. p. 292–9.
[148] Kutdede A, Sancak AA. Botulism in a long-legged buzzard (Buteo rutinus) [abstract]. Vet Rec 2002;151(2):64.
[149] Orr K. Botulism in a California condor (Gymnogyps californianus). Proc Am Assoc Zoo Vet 2002;101–3.
[150] St. Leger J, Reidarson T, Burch L. Managing avian botulism in California brown pelicans (Pelicanus occidentalis) [abstract]. Proc Assoc Avian Vet 2002;201.
[151] Kimura J. Electrodiagnosis in diseases of nerve and muscle: principles and practice. 2nd edition. Philadelphia: FA Davis Co.; 1993.
[152] Cuddon P. Electrophysiology in neuromuscular disease. Vet Clin North Am Small Anim Pract 2002;32(1):31–62.
[153] Shell L. Brachial plexus injury in two red-tailed hawks. J Wildl Dis 1993;29(1):177–9.
[154] Holland M, Jennings D. Use of electromyography in seven injured wild birds. J Am Vet Med Assoc 1997;211(5):607–9.
[155] Anderson RJ, Robertson DG, Henderson JD, et al. DFP-induced elevation of strength–duration threshold in hen peripheral nerve. Neurotoxicology 1988;9(1):47–52.
[156] Lidksy TI, Manetto C, Ehrich M. Nerve conduction studies in chickens given phenyl salignenin phosphate and corticosterone. J Toxicol Environ Health 1990;29(1):65–75.
[157] Massicotte C, Barber DS, Jornter BS, et al. Nerve conduction and ATP concentrations in sciatic–tibial and medial plantar nerves of hens given saligenin phospate. Neurotoxicology 2001;22(1):91–8.
[158] Robertson DG, Anderson RJ. Electrophysiologic characteristics of tibial and sciatic nerves in the hen. Am J Vet Res 1986;47(6):1378–81.
[159] Robertson DG, Mattson AM, Bestervelt LL, et al. Time course of electrophysiologic effects induced by di-n-butyl-2,2-dichlorovinyl phosphate (DBCV) in the adult hen. J Toxicol Environ Health 1988;23(3):283–94.
[160] Robertson DG, Schwab BW, Sills RD, et al. Electrophysiologic changes following treatment with organophosphorus-induced delayed neuropathy-producing agents in the adult hen. Toxicol Appl Pharmacol 1987;87(3):420–9.
[161] Shell L, Jortner BS, Ehrich M. Assessment of organophosphorous-induced delayed neuropathy in chickens using needle electromyography. J Toxicol Environ Health 1988; 24:21–33.
[162] Varhese RG. Organophosphorus-induced delayed neurotoxicity: a comparative study of the effects of Tri'ortho-tolyl phospahate and triphenyl phosphite on the central nervous system of the Japanese quail. Neurobehav Toxicol 1995;16(1):45–54.
[163] Lambert EH. Diagnostic value of electrical stimulation of motor nerves. Electroencephalogr Clin Neurophysiol 1962;22(Suppl):1–16.
[164] Maguire PJ, Smith MO, Wimsatt JH. Motor nerve conduction velcocity in the medianoulnar and sciatic/tibial nerves of pigeons [abstract]. J Vet Intern Med 1998;12(3):249.

[165] Kornegay JN, Gorgacz EJ, Parker MA, et al. Motor nerve conduction velocity in normal chickens. Am J Vet Res 1983;44:1537–40.

[166] Bagley RS, Wheeler SJ, James RL. Age-related effects on motor nerve conduction velocity in chickens. Am J Vet Res 1992;53:1309–11.

[167] Clippinger TL, Platt SR, Bennett RA, et al. Electrodiagnostic evaluation of peripheral nerve function in rheas and barred owls. Am J Vet Res 2000;61(4):469–72.

[168] Bagley RS, Wheeler SJ, Gay JM. Effects of age on temperature-related variation in motor nerve conduction velocity in healthy chickens. Am J Vet Res 1995;56(6):819–21.

[169] Campbell WW, Ward LC, Swift TR. Nerve conduction velocity varies inversely with height. Muscle Nerve 1981;3:436–7.

[170] Bagley RS, Wheeler SJ, James RL. Maturational changes in F waves in growing chickens. Am J Vet Res 1993;54(5):805–7.

[171] Dickinson PJ, LeCouteur RA. Muscle and nerve biopsy. Vet Clin North Am Small Anim Pract 2002;32(1):63–102.

[172] Bicknese EJ. Review of avian sarcocystosis. Proc Assoc Avian Vet 1993;52–8.

[173] Sutherland-Smith M, Morris P. Combination therapy using trimethoprim-sulfamethoxazole, pyrimethamine, and diclazuril to treat sarcocystosis in a pied imperial pigeon (Ducula bicolor bicolor). J Avian Med Surg 2004;18(3):151–4.

[174] Teglas MB, Little SE, Latimer KS, et al. Sarcocystis-associated encephalitis and myocarditis in a wild turkey (Meleagris gallopavo). J Parasitol 1998;84(3):661–3.

[175] Redding RW, Knecht CE. Atlas of electroencephalography in the dog and cat. New York: Praeger Special Studies; 1984.

[176] Pearson R. Electroencephalographic activity. The avian brain. London: Academic Press Inc.; Ltd., 1972. p. 564–89.

ELSEVIER
SAUNDERS

VETERINARY
CLINICS
Exotic Animal Practice

Vet Clin Exot Anim 10 (2007) 837–853

Reptilian Neurology: Anatomy and Function

Jeanette Wyneken, PhD

*Department of Biological Sciences, Building 01, Sanson Science, Florida Atlantic University,
777 Glades Road, Boca Raton, FL 33431-0991, USA*

The reptilian nervous system is moderately simple in structure yet allows great functional diversity in species-specific behaviors and adaptation to diverse niches. Although there is a certain amount of specialization of the nervous system of various reptilian species, it is more similar among reptile taxa than different. Superimposed upon these gross morphological and functional similarities are several significant variations that reflect differences in gross body structure and evolutionary history among turtles, snakes, lizards, crocodilians, and the tuatara.

The nervous system components

The components of the reptilian nervous system are defined as in other vertebrates. The reptilian central nervous system (CNS) includes the linearly organized brain and spinal cord. The peripheral nervous system (PNS) includes all nervous tissues and structures outside of the CNS. As in other vertebrates, axons that travel together in the CNS are nerve tracts, and axons in the PNS are nerves. Nerves entering or leaving the braincase are cranial nerves; those arising from or leaving the spinal cord are spinal nerves. Nerves carrying information to the CNS are sensory (afferent) nerves. Those carrying signals away from the CNS are motor (efferent) nerves. Peripheral nerves are classified as somatic motor (to skeletal muscle, etc.), somatic sensory (from skeletal muscle, integument, and related structures), visceral motor (to viscera, smooth muscle, cardiac muscle, and glands), or visceral sensory (from these same structures). Table 1 provides a summary of definitions of the key anatomical parts of the nervous system.

This work was supported in part by the National Marine Fisheries Service, contract to JW, and personal funds.

E-mail address: jwyneken@fau.edu

Table 1
Some definitions of parts of the cellular and multicellular parts of the nervous system

Neuron	Nerve cell
Nerve	Bundle of neurons or axons wrapped in connective tissue traveling together
Ganglion	Clusters of cell bodies of individual neurons
Sensory neuron (afferent neuron)	Transmits external stimuli from receptors toward central nervous system
Interneuron	Neuron found between sensory and motor neurons that integrates and relays signals
Motor neuron (efferent neuron)	Transmits signals to effector cells to provide responses
Cell body	The main part of neuron with cytoplasm, nucleus, and other organelles
Dendrites	Short outgrowths of cell body that carry signals to cell body
Axon	Long outgrowth of cell body that carry signals to next neuron or target cell
Dorsal root ganglion (spinal ganglion)	An enlarged part of the dorsal root that contains cell bodies of afferent spinal nerve neurons
Ventral root	Efferent somatic and visceral spinal nerve fibers
Propriospinal tract	Neurons that have the cell body in one spinal segment and axons terminating another spinal segment.
Cranial nerves	Axons of nerves entering or leaving brain; their dorsal and ventral roots are within the braincase and do not unite as in spinal nerves.

Definitions from Kardong K Vertebrates: comparative anatomy, function, evolution. 4th edition. Boston: WCB/McGraw-Hill; 2005 and Hyman LH. A laboratory manual for comparative vertebrate anatomy. Chicago: University of Chicago Press. 1942.

Gross anatomy of the central nervous system and landmarks

The reptilian CNS is tubular, organized linearly (Fig. 1), and has some degree of dorsoventral flexure along its length [1]. The brain is located mid-sagittally and is housed with in a tubular braincase bounded rostrally by the ethmoid cartilages, laterally by the otic bone series, ventrally by the basisphenoid and laterosphenoid, and caudally by the occipital bone series. The bones forming the midventral floor of the braincase also form the midline the roof of the mouth. The braincase is roofed by the supraoccipital, parietal, and frontal bones [2].

Reptiles have both subdural (beneath the dura mater) and epidural (above the dura mater) spaces within the brain case. There is substantial endocranial space between the brain and the roof and walls of the braincase in many lizards, aquatic turtles, and tuataras; there is moderate endocranial space in tortoises and crocodilians, and minimal endocranial space exists in snakes.

Reptiles have a poorly studied blood–brain barrier formed by the meninges, endothelial lining of the brain's blood supply, and the choroid plexus

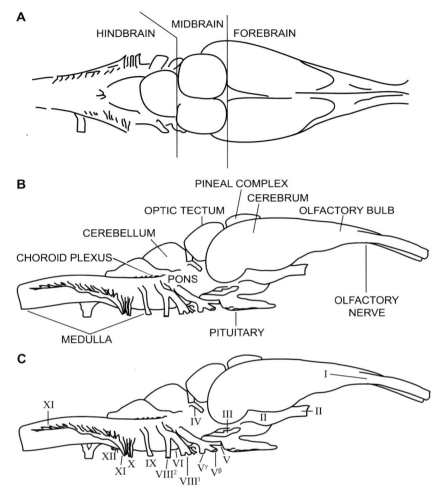

Fig. 1. Gross structure of a reptilian brain. This diagram is generalized from turtles and lizards. (*A*) Dorsal view showing major regions. (*B*) Lateral view with major external components identified. (*C*) The cranial nerves, labeled by Roman numerals, in a nonsquamate reptile. Rostral is toward the right.

[3]. The brain and spinal cord are surrounded by clear cerebrospinal fluid (CSF) that also fills the ventricles and the spinal cord's central canal. CSF is produced by the tela choroidea, a specialized vascular structure located in the dorsal midbrain. In lower vertebrates, the distal end of the central spinal canal, the terminal ventricle (ampulla caudalis), is the main site of CSF resorption into blood [4]. The spinal cord of reptiles extends virtually the entire length of the vertebral canal, continuing well into the tail. There is no cauda equina.

Two meninges cover the brain and spinal cord. The outer dura mater is tough and largely avascular; the inner leptomeninx is the more delicate, vascular and lies directly on the brain's surface [1]. There is no middle arachnoid mater or subarachnoid space. CSF is found between the dura mater and leptomeninx. The epidural space contains veins located ventral or lateral to the spinal cord. It does not contain CSF.

Brain development, form, and function

The brain develops as three large vesicles: the forebrain, midbrain, and hindbrain (see Fig. 1), which form early in development at the rostral end of the forming nerve tube. The forebrain is associated with smell, taste, rhythms, and sensory–motor integration and mediation. The midbrain is associated with visual processing and neuroendocrine roles. The hindbrain is associated with hearing, balance, and physiological homeostasis. External and internal landmarks roughly delineate these divisions. The forebrain is long and extends from the nose to the eyes; an imaginary line drawn between the eyes roughly identifies the caudal extent of the cerebrum and the optic chiasm in most reptiles [1]. The forebrain includes the lateral and third ventricles. The midbrain extends from the external landmarks of the eyes to the level of the ears. It is formed largely by the optic tectum (optic lobes) and tegmentum that surround the cerebral aqueduct. The hindbrain extends from the ear to the foramen magnum and includes the cerebellum, pons, medulla oblongata, tela choroidea, and fourth ventricle (see Fig. 1B). Each of these brain regions is subdivided further topographically and/or histologically into smaller subdivisions (Table 2).

The reptilian brain is roughly linear with some flexure between the midbrain and hindbrain [1]. When viewed dorsally (Fig. 2), the most rostral portions form the telencephalon and include the cerebrum and olfactory tracts, which lead caudally from the olfactory sacs to the olfactory bulbs. Immediately caudally are the relatively large paired cerebral hemispheres. Paired lobes of the mesencephalon, the tectum, follow next, then an unpaired cerebellum and other hind brain components (see Fig. 2, Table 2).

The olfactory sacs are perhaps the most rostral of the sensory structures innervated by cranial nerves. They are innervated by short olfactory nerves that run into long olfactory tracts, which project caudally to olfactory bulbs. Animals with elongated snouts (eg, alligators, monitor lizards, aquatic turtles) have long olfactory tracts [1] leading from the olfactory bulbs to the cerebrum.

The cerebral hemispheres include the pallium dorsally, and well-developed dorsal ventricular ridges internally and subpallium ventrally [2]; they lack the cortical folding (sulcus/gyrus structure) found in higher vertebrates. In most reptiles, the neocortex is absent; however, in chelonians, there is some evidence that the internal dorsal ventricular ridge is homologous to

Table 2
Reptilian brain divisions, subdivisions, and their components

Forebrain	Telencephalon	Olfactory tracts and bulbs; cerebral hemispheres; dorsal ventricular ridge; lateral ventricles; cranial nerve 0 (nervus terminalis); cranial nerve I (olfactory n)
Forebrain	Diencephalon	Hypothalamus and thalamus; dorsal thalamus and ventral thalamus; infundibulum and pituitary; pineal complex; optic chiasma; cranial nerves II (optic n) and III (oculomotor n)
Midbrain	Mesencephalon	Tectum (optic lobes); tegmentum; third ventricle; cerebral aqueduct; cranial nerve IV (trochlear n)
Hindbrain	Metencephalon	Cerebellum; anterior medulla; fourth ventricle; cranial nerves V (trigeminal n), VI (abducens n), VII (facial n), VIII (statoaccoustic n), IX (glossopharyngeal n), and X (vagus n)
Hindbrain	Myelencephalon	Medulla oblongata, cranial nerves XI (spinal accessory n) and XII (hypoglossal n)

Cranial nerves in these regions are noted by the positions from which they arise from the brain and not their paths or targets. The brain stem includes the mesencephalon and metencephalon.
Abbreviation: n, nerve.

the neocortex of mammals [5]. The cerebral hemispheres receive olfactory information directly and process other sensory information from the thalamus.

The pineal complex (epiphysis and the parietal eye) arises just caudal to the cerebrum by means of a thin stalk; it extends to the dorsal skull at the region of the pineal scale (when present [6,7]) and is responsible for regulating pigmentation and biological rhythms. The epiphysis or pineal gland is located deep to the pineal eye scale in iguanine lizards and *Sphenodon* and deep to the pink spot of leatherback sea turtles (*Dermochelys coriacea*). In other taxa, its position is not demarked by an external landmark as clearly. The pineal gland is both sensory and secretory and is important in regulating circadian rhythms in many animals. It is not well-developed in snakes and crocodilians [2].

The tectum is composed of paired (optic) lobes located caudal to the cerebral hemispheres. The tectum receives both visual and auditory input. The size of the tectum is correlated with the importance of visual stimuli to the animal [2,8].

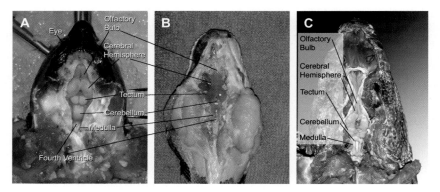

Fig. 2. Dorsal views of the brain in (*A*) a freshwater turtle (*Trachemys scripta*), (*B*) a boa constrictor (*Boa constrictor*), and (*C*) a green iguana (*Iguana iguana*) showing the major dorsal structures of the brain.

Generally, reptiles hear lower frequencies. Auditory processing centers are located in the medulla oblongata, cerebellum, and parts of the tectum and the thalamus. Relatively few detailed studies of auditory processing are available for reptiles, perhaps because so few species appear to use airborne sound (the exceptions may be the geckos (eg, *Gecko gecko*) and crocodilians (eg, *Alligator mississippiensis*). Statoacoustic nerves from each cochlea project unilaterally to several nuclei in the midbrain. Projections from these auditory processing tracts become bilateral in the hindbrain. The details of reptile auditory anatomy are summarized elsewhere [9–12].

The cerebellum, part of the hind brain, is a single structure that integrates touch, proprioception, vision, hearing, and motor input and has a role in maintaining postural equilibrium. It is organized and functions similarly in all vertebrates [13]. As in mammals and birds, it is important in coordinating and modifying motor actions. Cerebellar size varies among species and particularly with locomotor behavior; it tends to be smaller in ground-dwelling species and larger in aquatic and climbing species. Structurally the reptile cerebellum is formed by a large corpus cerebelli and small flocculus. The corpus cerebelli is divided into three anatomical and functional regions [13–15]. In turtles, one region is thicker and associated with the restriction of locomotor movements in the legs. A different region of the corpus cerebelli is thicker in animals that use axial muscles in locomotion (snakes and legless lizards). The crocodilian cerebellum is larger and structurally more complex than in other reptiles, with two transverse sulci separating it into three lobes [13,15].

The medulla oblongata portion of the hindbrain is fairly conservative and appears to function as in other vertebrates. It houses the visceral, auditory, proprioceptive, and respiratory centers; controls basic heart rate; and regulates gastrointestinal mobility and secretion [2].

Cranial nerves

Cranial nerves are part of the PNS but will be discussed here with other cranial structures. They are formed by peripheral axons and control many of the vital functions of the body. The functions of most can be evaluated in reptiles. Caudal to the olfactory nerve and nervus terminalis nerves, the remaining cranial nerves emerge ventrally and laterally from the brain. There are 12 to 13 cranial nerves in most reptiles (Fig. 1C; Table 3), but just 11 to 12 in snakes. The terminal nerves (nervus terminalis, cranial nerve 0) travel with the olfactory nerves; the two are the most rostral cranial nerves. It was discovered in lower vertebrates after the classical naming (human-based) and numbering system was in place. Its study in reptiles is limited; the terminal nerve function remains unclassified; however, it believed to be associated with one or more gonadotropin-releasing hormones (GnRH) as in other lower vertebrates [7,16,17]. Its function cannot be tested clinically under most circumstances. The terminal nerve innervates the vasculature of the nasal epithelium. The locations and functions of the cranial nerves of reptiles are summarized in Fig. 2 and Tables 2 and 3. In groups of animals that lack legs, the spinal accessory nerve is reduced or absent [7,18,19]. Most cranial nerve functions can be tested (see Table 3).

Visual system

Retinal ganglion cells communicate signals from the receptors (rods and/ or cones) to brain; their axons form the optic nerves, an extension of the brain; the optic nerves converge in the optic chiasma. These nerve tracts primarily project to the contralateral side of the optic tectum but also may have limited ipsilateral projections in turtles, snakes and lizards; *Sphenodon* and crocodilians lack ipsilateral nerve tract components [20]. The ipsilateral projections are related to binocular vision in mammals, but reptiles may have binocular vision without ipsilateral projections. The major visual centers receiving optic synapses are located in the hypothalamus. Several centers are located in the thalamus and pretectum, superficial layers of the optic tectum, and in the nucleus opticus tegmenti [20]. The snake visual neuroanatomy differs in structural organization from that in other reptiles, perhaps because of the importance of their other sensory systems (infrared pit organs and the vomeronasal organ) or even because of their phylogenetic history. Snake nerve tract projections to the superficial tectum are absent or organized into fewer layers with less complexity than in other reptiles [20].

Olfactory and vomeronasal systems

Olfactory nerves travel by means of the olfactory tracts to the olfactory cortex of the telencephalon. In at least lizards and snakes, a tract from

Table 3
Reptilian cranial nerves, their function and clinical tests to detect neurological anomalies

Nerve	Function	Clinical test
0 Nervus terminalis	Innervates vasculature of nasal epithelium; chemosensory for GnRH	None
I Olfactory (including the vomeronasal [VNO] nerve branch)	Olfaction, carries sensory information from the nasal sacs and VNO	Patient should avoid noxious odor such as alcohol, or orient toward food when eyes are covered
II Optic	Vision, carries sensory information from the retina to the thalamus and optic tectum	Check menace response in patients with eyelids and reaction to threatening movement.
III Oculomotor	Controls movement of eye; tends to pull eye in or fix gaze; controls iris and ciliary body	Check for normal, coordinated eye movement; check pupillary light reflex and pupil shape.
IV Trochlear	Controls movement of eye; draws gaze anteriorly and dorsally	Look for normal, coordinated eye movement (includes cranial nerves VI and VII); check for strabismus.
V Trigeminal three branches: ophthalmic, maxillary, and mandibular nerves	Sensory from skin around eye and mouth. Sensory pits of pit vipers and boids. Controls jaw adductor muscles, muscles of skin around teeth-bearing bones in snakes, and intermandibularis (in floor of mouth).	Mandibular branch: check normal jaw closure and buccal pumping. Ophthalmic branch and maxillary branch: test patient's ability to feel stimulus to face, lower lid, and nasal area
VI Abducens	Controls movement of eye, draws gaze posteriorly	Look for normal, coordinated eye movement (includes cranial nerves IV and VI); check for strabismus
VII Facial	Sensory from skin and muscle around the ear, upper jaw, and pharynx. Controls superficial neck muscles and mandibular depressor.	Normal movement of lids in patients with lids. Patient should be able to open mouth voluntarily (if compliant).
VIII Statoacoustic = acoustic = auditory	Balance and hearing: sensory from the inner ear	Turn head left and right to check for brief and spontaneous nystagmus; check for defect such as head tilt, atypical posture, poor righting reflex. Audiograms are of questionable value as auditory range is documented poorly in many species.

(continued on next page)

Table 3 (*continued*)

Nerve	Function	Clinical test
IX Glossopharyngeal	Taste and sensation in the pharynx; controls tongue muscles	Examine tongue for active protrusion and retraction. Observe ability to swallow.
X Vagus	Sensory and motor to glottis, heart, and viscera	Apply pressure to both eyes for several minutes and check for decreased heart rate. Observe ability to swallow, opening and closing glottis.
XI Spinal accessory	Controls trapezius and sternomastoid muscles	Dorsal neck and shoulder muscles should have strong tone in lizards and crocodilians; difficult to assess in snakes (if present) and in turtles.
XII Hypoglossal	Controls hyoid muscles and tongue.	Look for deviation of the tongue to indicate defects.

Adapted from Chrisman C, Walsh M, Meeks JC, et al. Neurologic examination is sea turtles. J Am Vet Med Assoc 1997;211(8):1043–7 and J Wyneken and DR Mader. 2005, ARAV focus lectures, Reptilian Neurology: Anatomy, Function and Clinical Applications, Tucson, Arizona, 10–14 April 2005.)

the vomeronasal organ also projects to the cerebrum by means of an accessory olfactory tract. The terminal nerve (nervus terminalis) innervates the nasal septum; its ganglion is associated with gonadotropin-releasing hormone [7,21,22].

Vestibulocochlear system

As in other vertebrates, the vestibulocochlear system detects sound or vibrations through the auditory apparatus (columella and inner ear structures) and movement and orientation in space [2]. Auditory nerves from each lagena (equivalent to the cochlea of mammals) project to the auditory tectum. The vestibular apparatus (semicircular canals, sacculus, and utriculus) is innervated by branches of the statoacoustic (= auditory = acoustic = vestibulocochlear) nerve that process information in the medulla. Generally, reptiles hear lower frequencies and detect seismic vibrations [2].

Spinal cord

The spinal cord travels in the spinal canal of the vertebral column, often with one or more veins. The cord generally fills only a portion of the canal, with more than 50% of the lumen free in alligators and 29% to 34% free in several lizards species [23]. The spinal cord is organized segmentally as in

other vertebrates with the cranial-most segments controlling or receiving signals from the more cranial structures. The cord tends to be larger toward the
brain associated with the greater numbers of nerve tracts traveling to or
from lower spinal segments along side tracks to or from more cranial segments. The reptilian spinal cord lacks some of the functional regionalization
seen in higher vertebrates. Because of the tremendous variation in vertebral
segment number among taxa and the lack of distinct regional boundaries,
spinal segments typically are numbered from the first cervical segment on
caudally. The cord is enlarged in cross section in the cervical and sacral regions corresponding to the brachial and sacral plexuses (also termed lumbosacral plexus, although reptiles lack a lumbar region) (Fig. 3) [24–26] in
turtles, lizards, and crocodilians. In snakes, the cord is expanded in the midtrunk [27].

The spinal cord has outer white matter surrounding internal gray matter
that is organized as dorsal and ventral horns (Fig. 4). The white matter is
formed of myelinated axons and connects the brainstem to the rest of the
cord by means of long bundles of ascending and descending nerve fibers.
The gray matter, formed of cell bodies, varies relatively little in total

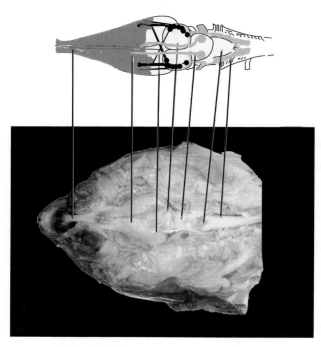

Fig. 3. Dorsal view and diagram of brain in a turtle (*Trachemys scripta*) diagrammatically the
major sensory processing regions of the olfactory processing regions are shown in dark gray;
visual processing regions are black, and auditory processing regions are shown in light gray.
After [9,24–26].

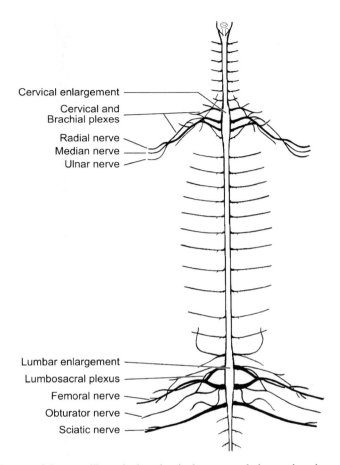

Fig. 4. Diagram of the a reptilian spinal cord, spinal nerves, and plexuses based on an alligator (*Alligator mississippiensis*). *Modified after* Reese AM. The alligator and its allies. New York: G. Putmanls Sons; 1915 and Hildebrand M. Analysis of vertebrate structure. New York: John Wiley & Sons, Inc. 1974.

cross-sectional area along the length of the cord in lizards and turtles, although the extent of the dorsal and ventral roots varies along the cranial to caudal axis [27–29]. Reptiles have collateral branching of axons in the descending propriospinal fibers [28].

The gray matter in the spinal cord of reptiles is organized into bilaterally symmetrical dorsal and ventral horns. The dorsal horns include dorsal roots, and the ventral horns have motor neurons. The ventral horns are reduced in the midtrunk of tortoises (and probably other turtles), presumably because of fewer motor neurons associated with the lack of trunk musculature. Between the dorsal and ventral horns is a large area of gray matter formed of interneurons [28].

Spinal nerves

The PNS includes laterally paired spinal nerves (see Fig. 4) that arise from the spinal cord as dorsal and ventral nerve roots; these nerves then exit the vertebrae by means of intervertebral foramina. The number of spinal nerve pairs is a function of vertebral number, so snakes often have far more spinal nerves than other reptilian species [28]. The dorsal roots are composed primarily of somatic and visceral sensory nerve fibers but may contain motor fibers also; the ventral roots are composed of both somatic and visceral motor nerve fibers in reptiles (Fig. 5) [8].

The visceral nerves function as the autonomic nervous system (ANS) with both sympathetic and parasympathetic components. The basic ANS pattern is a preganglionic nerve fiber whose cell body is in the CNS and whose axon synapses with a peripheral nerve that innervates the target tissue [2]. Beyond this pattern, the reptilian ANS differs from that of mammals in that the autonomic visceral nerves are not anatomically segregated into thoraco–lumbar sympathetic and cranio–sacral parasympathetic regions. In reptiles, the autonomic visceral nerves arise along the length of the spinal

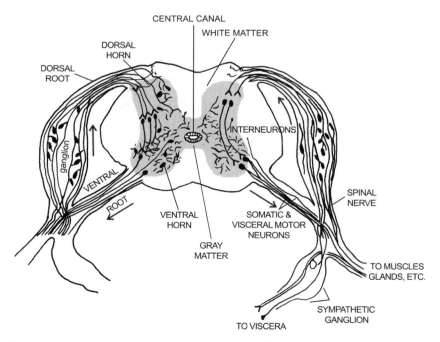

Fig. 5. Diagrammatic spinal cord cross section is generalized from cross sections of the cord and spinal nerves of an alligator (*Alligator mississippiensis*), black tegu (*Tupinambis nigropunctatus*), red ear slider (*Trachemys scripta*), and an unidentified snake. The spinal cord is organized as the white matter and gray matter, although the color margins are often not as distinct as in mammals. Reptile spinal nerves are organized as dorsal and ventral roots.

cord and may have both sympathetic and parasympathetic components [29]. The sympathetic nerves form a short chain of ganglia adjacent to the vertebral column, with long postganglionic fibers running to the viscera. The ANS anatomy is understood mostly from studies of lizards [8].

The sympathetic nervous system has bilateral sympathetic ganglia (sympathetic trunks). Preganglionic fibers are myelinated and emerge segmentally in truck region between the limb plexuses. The postganglionic fibers are unmyelinated and synapse with the sympathetic trunk along the entire length of the body. The more rostral preganglionic fibers innervate the heart, lungs, and more cranial viscera, while the middle and more caudal fibers innervate the alimentary canal, peripheral blood vessels, chromatophores (in some lizards), spleen, and urogenital system [8].

The sympathetic neurotransmitter is primarily norepinephrine (noradrenalin). However, epinephrine (adrenalin) stimulates contraction in the reproductive systems of some lizards [30,31], and some cholinergic fibers are found there also [31]. Sympathetic stimulation is the fight-or-flight response that increases visceral activity (while slowing digestion), metabolism, heart rate, dilates pulmonary vasculature and causes adrenal secretion [8,32]. It is unclear if pupil dilation is under sympathetic control in reptiles [8].

Parasympathetic stimulation is cholinergic (acetylcholine release) in reptiles as in higher vertebrates, and restores the resting state by constricting lungs, slowing heart rate, allowing metabolism to return to normal. Vagal innervation of the visceral muscles, stomach, and lungs is under adrenergic inhibitory control. Vagal innervation of the reptilian heart is by means of separate parasympathetic inhibitory cholinergic fibers and adrenergic cardioaccelerator fibers [31].

Spinal reflexes

Spinal reflexes are part of reptilian nervous system control. Somatic spinal reflexes sense and control muscles, tendons, and skin to maintain posture. Visceral spinal reflexes control cardiac muscle, smooth muscles of the digestive tract and blood vessels, and glands [2]. Spinal reflexes are important in clinical assessment of reptile patients [33,34].

Plexuses

Two networks of interconnected spinal nerves are associated with control of the limbs: the cervical or brachial plexus and the sacral (or lumbosacral) plexus (see Fig. 4) [35,36]. Snakes, because of the absence of limbs, either lack or have reduced brachial and sacral plexuses [37–39]. Plexuses are formed by ventral nerve roots and their branches. The brachial plexus arises from the more caudal cervical spinal nerves. These cervical nerves form a complex network innervating shoulder and forelimb muscles and may send branches to the respiratory muscles. Most muscles receive innervation from more than one branch of the plexus. The cervical plexus typically includes the median nerve and inferior brachial nerve. The latter divides to form the superficial radial nerve and the deep radial nerve to the shoulder and dorsal forelimb. The supracoracoideus, subscapular, and ulnar nerves innervate the pectoral muscles, subscapularis, and ventral forelimb muscles, while the deltoideus nerve innervates the shoulder [40–42].

The sacral plexus arises as four to six branches from spinal nerves associated with the last trunk vertebra and sacral vertebrae [40–42]. These nerves divide, and parts interconnect several times as nerves pass to the inguinal, pelvic, and hind limb muscles. Many muscles receive multiple innervations. The more caudal nerve roots give rise to the obturator nerve to the ventral pelvic muscles, and the ischiadicus nerve, which runs to the muscles of the ilium and then divides to form the peroneal and sciatic nerves. The more cranial nerve roots interconnect to provide major innervations (via crural, femoral, and tibial nerves) to the inguinal muscles, thigh adductors, and leg extensors [42]. There are also sacral branches going to the bladder. Sacral nerves are presumed to innervate the genitalia [41].

Basic nerve function

Nerves communicate with each other and with their target tissues by means of electrical signals and chemical signals (neurotransmitters) that diffuse across synapses. Neurotransmitters elicit an electrical response from the next neuron and are either excitatory or inhibitory. As in other vertebrates, the neurotransmitters include excitatory amino acids (glutamate, aspartate, and substance P [a peptide]), and acetylcholine in neuromuscular junctions [43,44]. Major inhibitory neurotransmitters include: catecholamines and indolamines such as dopamine, norepinepherine, epinephrine, GABA, glycine, taurine, and endorphin [43,45]. Acetylcholine also may function as an inhibitor when it binds to muscarinic ACh receptors associated with heart muscle [44,45]. Neurotransmitters in reptiles have not been fully studied; however, similar forms of neuropeptides share similar roles in many vertebrates [31,43]. This similarity may serve as a basis to anticipate how neurotransmitters might interact with common drugs and/or create toxic side effects.

Summary

The CNS is formed of the brain and spinal cord.

The brain is longitudinally organized and tubular. Its surface is typically smooth.

The brain has neuroendocrine components (pineal, hypophysis).

The details of nerve tracts leading into or away from the brain differ among taxa, yet the gross structure of the brain is similar among reptiles.

The CNS's architecture includes gray matter (with little or no myelin) and white matter (myelinated axons). In the spinal cord, the gray matter is internal to the white matter, but is not always as distinct as in birds and mammals.

Gray matter is organized as dorsal and ventral roots. The size of the ventral roots diminishes in species that lack trunk musculature or do not use the axial body in locomotion.

The spinal cord extends the length of the body from the neck through the tail in reptiles. In chelonians, the spinal cord is housed within (neural) carapace bones from cervical vertebra 8 to the sacrum, and is contained within the spinal canal of free cervical, sacral, and caudal vertebrae that are not incorporated into the carapace.

The number of spinal segments differs with body form (many in snakes, few in turtles).

Cervical and sacral (lumbosacral) enlargements of the spinal cord are found in species with extremities.

The PNS is all nervous tissue outside of CNS, including cranial nerves and spinal nerves.

The nervous system is divided into voluntary versus autonomic control.

The autonomic system is associated with most of the length of the spinal cord and is not partitioned regionally as in mammals.

Transmission of stimuli between neurons is by means of neurotransmitters at synapses. Neurotransmitters included in autonomic systems act antagonistically.

Neurotransmitter form and function often are inferred from mammalian systems.

Excitatory neurotransmitters include glutamate, aspirate, substance P, and acetylcholine in neuromuscular junctions; inhibitory neurotransmitters include dopamine, norepinepherine, epinephrine, GABA, glycine, taurine, and endorphins. Acetylcholine may be inhibitory when acting on membrane-bound muscarinic ACh receptors in heart muscle.

References

[1] Starck D. Craniocerebral relations in recent reptiles. In: C Gans, RG Northcutt, P Ulinski, editors. Biology of the reptilia. 1979. vol. 9 (Neurology A). New York: Academic Press. p. 1–38

[2] Kardong K. Vertebrates: comparative anatomy, function, evolution. 4th edition. Boston: WCB/McGraw-Hill; 2005.

[3] Cserr HF, Bundgaard M. Blood–brain interfaces in vertebrates: a comparative approach. Am J Physiol Regul Integr Comp Physiol 1984;246:277–88.

[4] Pérez-Fígares JM, Jimenez AJ, Rodríguez EM. Subcommissural organ, cerebrospinal fluid circulation, and hydrocephalus In: EM Rodríguez, CR Yulis, editors. Special issue: the subcommissural organ. Cellular, molecular, physiological and pathological aspects. Microscopy research and technique. 2001;52(5):591–607.

[5] Belekhova MG. Neurophysiology of the forebrain. In: Gans C, Northcutt RG, Ulinski P, editors. Biology of the reptilia. vol. 10 (Neurology B). Chicago: University of Chicago Press; 1979. p. 287–332.

[6] Quay WB. The parietal eye-pineal complex. In: Gans C, Northcutt RG, Ulinski P, editors. Biology of the reptilia. Chicago: University of Chicago Press; 1979. vol. 9 (Neurology A). p. 245–406.

[7] Jacobson E. Infectious diseases and pathology in reptiles: color atlas and text. Boca Raton, Florida: CRC/Taylor and Frances Press; 2007.

[8] Berger PJ, Burnstock G. Autonomic nervous system. In: Gans C, Northcutt RG, Ulinski P, editors. Biology of the reptilia. vol. 10 (Neurology B). Chicago: University of Chicago Press; 1979. p. 1–57.

[9] Carr CE, Code RA. The central auditory system of reptiles and birds. In: Dooling RJ Fay RR, Popper A, editors. Comparative hearing: birds and reptiles. New York: Springer; 2000. p. 197–248.

[10] Dooling RJ, Lohr B, Dent ML. Hearing in birds and reptiles. In: Dooling RJ, Fay RR, Popper A, editors. Comparative hearing: birds and reptiles. New York: Springer; 2000. p. 308–60.

[11] Manley GA. Evolution of structure and function of the hearing organ of lizards. J Neurobiol 2002;53:202–11.

[12] Wever EG. The reptile ear. Princeton (NJ): Princeton Univ. Press; 1978.

[13] ten Donklelaar HJ, Bangma GC. The cerebellum. In: Gans C, Ulinski P, editors. Biology of the reptilia. vol. 17 (Neurology C). Chicago: University of Chicago Press; 1992. p. 497–586.

[14] Larsell O. The cerebellum of reptiles: lizards and snakes. J Comp Neurol 1926;41:59–94.

[15] Larsell O. The cerebellum of reptiles: chelonians and alligator. J Comp Neurol 1932;56: 59–94.

[16] Demski LS. Terminal nerve complex. Acta Anat 1993;148(2–3):81–95.

[17] Nieuwenhuys R, ten Donkelaar HJ, Nicholson C. The central nervous system of vertebrates. New York: Springer; 1998.

[18] Huxley TH. A manual of the anatomy of vertebrate animals. New York: D. Appleton and Company; 1881.

[19] Hinsey JC. The functional components of the dorsal roots of spinal nerves. Q Rev Biol 1933; 8(4):457–64.

[20] Repérant J, Rio J-P, Ward RS, et al. Comparative analysis of the visual system of reptiles. In: Gans C, Ulinski P, editors. Biology of the reptilia. vol. 17. Neurology C, Sensory Motor Integration. Chicago: University of Chicago Press; 1992. p. 175–240.

[21] Skeen LC, Pindzola RR, Schofield BR. Tangential organization of olfactory, association, and commissural projections to olfactory cortex in a species of reptile (Trionyx spiniferus), bird (Aix sponsa), and mammal (Tupaia glis). Brain Behav Evol 1984;25(4):206–16.

[22] Smeets JAJ, Hoogland V, Lohman AHM. A forebrain atlas of the lizard Gecko gecko. J Comp Neurol 1986;254(1):1–19.

[23] Giffin EB. Functional interpretation of spinal anatomy in vertebrate paleontology. In: Thomason JJ, editor. Functional morphology in vertebrate paleontology; Cambridge: Cambridge University Press; 1995. p. 235–48.

[24] Huber GC, Crosby EC. The reptilian optic tectum. J Comp Neurol 1933;57(1):57–163.

[25] ten Donkelaar HJ, Nieuwenhuys R. The brainstem. In: Gans C, Northcutt RG, Ulinski P, editors. Biology of the reptilia. vol. 10 (Neurology B). Chicago: University of Chicago Press; 1979. p. 133–200.

[26] Scwab EM. Variation in the rhombencephalon. In: Gans C, Northcutt RG, Ulinski P, editors. Biology of the reptilia. Chicago: University of Chicago Press; 1979. vol. 10 (Neurology B). p. 200–46.

[27] Kusuma A, ten Donkelaar HJ, Nieuwenhuys R. Intrinsic organization of the spinal cord. In: Gans C, Northcutt RG, Ulinski P, editors. Biology of the reptilia. Chicago: University of Chicago Press; 1979. vol. 10 (Neurology B). p. 59–109.

[28] Kusuma A, ten Donkelaar HJ. Propriospinal fibers interconnecting the spinal enlargements in some quadrupedal reptiles. J Comp Neurol 1980;193(4):871–91.

[29] Cruce WLR. Spinal cord in lizards. In: Gans C, Northcutt RG, Ulinski P, editors. Biology of the reptilia. Chicago: University of Chicago Press; 1979. vol. 10 (Neurology B). p. 111–31.

[30] Zurich L, Paz De La Vega-Lemus Y, Lemus D. Presence of adrenergic receptors in the uterus of two species of lizards, *Liolaemus gravenhorfi* and *Liolaemus tenuis* tenuis. Biol Reprod 1971;5:123–6.

[31] Burnstock G. Evolution of the autonomic innervation of visceral and cardiovascular systems in vertebrates. Pharmacol Rev 1969;21:247–324.

[32] Crossley DA II, Wang T, Altimiras J. Role of nitric oxide in the systemic and pulmonary circulation of anesthetized turtles (*Trachemys scripta*). J Exp Zool 2000;286:683–9.

[33] Bennett RA, Mehler SJ. Neurology. In: Mader DR, editor. Reptile medicine and surgery. St. Louis (MO): Elsevier; 2006. p. 239–50.

[34] Chrisman C, Walsh M, Meeks JC, et al. Neurologic examination is sea turtles. J Am Vet Med Assoc 1997;211(8):1043–7.

[35] Reese AM. The alligator and its allies. New York: G. Putman's Sons; 1915.

[36] Hildebrand M. Analysis of vertebrate structure. New York: John Wiley & Sons, Inc; 1974.

[37] Goodrich ES. Memoirs: metameric segmentation and homology. Q J Microsc Sci 1913; s2–59:227–8.

[38] Owen R. The anatomy of vertebrates, vol. 1: Fishes and Reptiles. London: Longmans, Green, and Co; 1866.

[39] Edlinger L. The anatomy of the central nervous system of man and vertebrates in general. Philadelphia: The F.A. Davis Publisher; 1899.

[40] Romer AS, Parsons TS. The vertebrate body. New York: Saunders College Publishing; 1986.

[41] Wyneken J. Guide to the anatomy of sea turtles. NMFS Tech. Publication; Miami: NOAA Tech., Memo NMFS-SEFSC-470. 2001

[42] Hyman LH. A laboratory manual for comparative vertebrate anatomy. Chicago: University of Chicago Press; 1942.

[43] Reiner A. Neuropeptides in the nervous system. In: Gans C, Ulinski P, editors. Biology of the reptilia. vol. 17. Neurology C, sensory motor integration. Chicago: University of Chicago Press; 1992. p. 587–739.

[44] Granda AM, Sisson DF. Retinal function if turtles. In: Gans C, Ulinski P, editors. Biology of the reptilia. vol. 17 (Neurology C). Chicago: University of Chicago Press; 1992. p. 136–73.

[45] Milton SL. The structure and function of the turtle brain: adaptations for resistance to anoxia. In: Wyneken J, Godfrey M, Bels V, editors. The biology of turtles. Boca Raton: CRC Press/Taylor & Francis Group, in press.

VETERINARY
CLINICS
Exotic Animal Practice

ELSEVIER
SAUNDERS

Vet Clin Exot Anim 10 (2007) 855–891

The Neurologic Examination and Neurodiagnostic Techniques for Reptiles

Christopher L. Mariani, DVM, PhD

*Department of Clinical Sciences, College of Veterinary Medicine,
North Carolina State University, 4700 Hillsborough Street,
Raleigh, NC 27606-1428, USA*

Living reptile species have been classified into four different orders: the *Chelonia* (turtles and tortoises), the *Rhynchocephalia* (consisting only of the tuatara [*Sphenodon*]), the Squamata (amphisbaenians, lizards and snakes), and the *Crocodilia* (alligators and crocodiles). Reptiles also may be classified in other ways, including a locomotion-based scheme. This distinguishes the *Lepidosauria* (tuatara, lizards, and snakes), which retain a sprawling posture, mediolateral movement of the limbs, and sinusoidal movements of the trunk (lateral undulation), from the *Archosauria* (alligators and dinosaurs), which reduce or eliminate lateral flexure of the vertebral column and have the limbs more directly beneath the body [1].

Although most veterinarians are familiar with performing neurologic examinations in companion animals such as dogs, cats, and horses, the prospect of evaluating a reptilian patient with a suspected neurologic disease can be daunting, because of profound differences in anatomy and physiology, and a dearth of knowledge concerning the normal biology of these animals. Many of the principles and techniques employed for mammalian patients can be adapted for use in reptiles, however, and can provide useful information to the practitioner deciding how to manage these cases [2–5].

The goal of the neurologic examination in any patient is to answer four main questions:

1. Is the problem arising from the nervous system?
2. If the problem is neurological, what is the location of the lesion?
3. What is the differential diagnosis?
4. How severe is the problem/What is the prognosis?

E-mail address: chris_mariani@ncsu.edu

doi:10.1016/j.cvex.2007.04.004   *vetexotic.theclinics.com*

856 MARIANI

The neurologic examination in veterinary patients traditionally has consisted of numerous tests, grouped as follows:

- Evaluation of mentation, awareness, and responsiveness
- Gait evaluation
- Cranial nerve examination
- Assessment of posture and postural reactions
- Assessment of segmental spinal reflexes
- Assessment of discomfort or pain (physiologic or pathologic)
- Assessment of muscle size and tone

The anatomy of various reptile species may render the performance of some of these tests difficult or impossible. In addition, in the case of dangerous animals (such as venomous snakes and large constrictors or monitor lizards), examination may be impossible without restraint or anesthesia. As a result, observation of the animal as it moves about its enclosure and interacts with its environment is a particularly important part of the examination. As reptiles are ectothermic, it is important that the examination take place at appropriate environmental temperatures, as low temperatures may result in reduced nerve conduction, weakness, sluggishness, behavioral changes, or frank neurologic deficits [4]. Each species has a preferred optimal temperature range (POTR), and knowledge of this range will help to ensure accurate examination results.

A detailed description of anatomic pathways and their functional correlates as assessed by the neurologic examination is beyond the scope of this article. Instead, the focus will be on specifics of performing the neurologic examination and neurodiagnostic testing in reptiles, and how these examinations differ from those performed in more conventional species. For a detailed description of neuroanatomy and neurologic examinations in companion animals, the reader is referred to other excellent sources of this information [6–8].

History and assessment of husbandry

As many diseases in reptiles, including neurologic conditions, are related to inadequate husbandry, a knowledge of proper environmental and dietary care for the species in question is imperative [4,9–13]. Information regarding these conditions is obtained through examination of the animal's enclosure, if available, and through questioning of the animal's owner or caretaker. Important factors to consider include the temperature range and gradient of the enclosure or environment, the diet and any supplements, the bedding, antibiotic, antiparasitic, or any other administered medications, the source of the animal, and the health of other animals in the collection.

Exposure to excessively low temperatures during hibernation or sudden drops in water temperature may result in neurologic abnormalities in chelonians [2,5,12,14–17]. Reptiles fed low-calcium diets may develop nutritional hyperparathyroidism, leading to tremors, muscle fasciculations, tetany, seizures, osteopenia, and possible fractures [2,12,18–21]. Thiamine deficiency may result from feeding fish-based diets (particularly frozen fish) to crocodilians, aquatic snakes, or chelonians, and may result in seizures, altered mentation, paresis, dysphagia, and vestibular signs [4,5,22,23]. Vitamin A deficiency can lead to squamous metaplasia of the tympanic cavity, particularly in chelonians, predisposing to bacterial infection and aural abscessation [24–26]. Feeding egg-based diets can result in biotin deficiency, while leaf-based diets from deficient soils can lead to vitamin E or selenium deficiency [2,4,14,27]. High-fat diets have been associated with the development of cholesterol granulomas (xanthomas) within the central nervous system (CNS) [4]. Intoxications leading to neurologic signs may result from improper bedding material (eg, wood shavings) [28], the ingestion of rhubarb [4,12], azalea [4], lead-based sinkers or paint [4,29], ethylene glycol [14], or animals such as *Bufo* toads [12,30]. Neurologic signs also may occur following treatment with chlorhexidine [31], aminoglycosides (weakness caused by neuromuscular blockade) [4,12,32,33], metronidazole (CNS signs) [4,12,15,34], enrofloxacin (hyperexcitability, incoordination) [35], ivermectin (stupor, coma, paresis) [2,15,36–39], organophosphates (eg, dichlorvos strips) [4,5,12,30], or other antiparasitic drugs.

As with conventional companion animals, it is imperative to include questions regarding inappetence, regurgitation, coughing, or other signs of illness, which may indicate involvement of other organ systems, or may suggest a potential etiology.

Neurologic examination

Mentation, awareness, and responsiveness

Mentation and responsiveness are indications of an animal's level of consciousness, which can be described on a graded scale as follows:

- Alert (normal and aware of surroundings)
- Obtunded (less aware and less responsive to surroundings, responds to stimuli)
- Stupor (even less aware and less responsive to stimuli, but will respond to noxious stimuli)
- Coma (unaware and unresponsive even to noxious stimuli)

Most reptiles are obviously alert and aware of their environment and will respond appropriately to opening of an enclosure, attempts to handle them, prodding with a pole or stick, offering of food, loud noises, or noxious stimuli such as poking with a needle or pinching with hemostats. For example, most lizards are quite alert, and try to escape when attempts are made to capture them [33,40,41]. Some species, however, are normally less animated, and seem less responsive to their environment (eg, crocodilians). Thus, the normal behavior of the species in question must be borne in mind [33,41,42]. Some species (eg, hog-nosed snakes) may feign death when threatened, and other normal behaviors such as tail displays, caudal luring, tonic immobility, and circumduction (arm waving) may mimic neurologic disease [42].

Abnormal behaviors such as frantic movement around an enclosure, walking into corners, walking in circles, head pressing, or inappropriate feeding behaviors that may be classified best as dementia or delirium may be observed, and suggest forebrain dysfunction. Reduced consciousness suggests an intracranial lesion, although severe systemic disease also may result in a moribund state and altered mentation, and must be ruled out. Evidence of seizures, tetany, or other abnormal movements should be recorded. It is worth noting that some species (eg, lizards and crocodilians) normally may enter a state of apparent stupor or hypnosis when a vasovagal maneuver is performed (eg, exerting ocular pressure) or when the animal is turned over and stroked on the abdomen. This often is used to the clinician's advantage for physical examination or to complete minor procedures such as radiography [9].

Gait examination

Things to evaluate during the gait examination include the presence of ataxia, paresis or weakness, and lameness. Whereas ataxia always indicates neurologic dysfunction, weakness also may be seen with muscle disease or a systemic illness. Lameness is often indicative of an orthopedic problem, but may be a manifestation of neurologic disease, particularly in cases of nerve or nerve root entrapment.

Gait examination is facilitated by providing an appropriate surface for the animal to move upon. Many reptiles will have difficulty moving on a stainless steel table, and a rougher surface (eg, thin blanket, bedding in enclosure) should be provided. Arboreal species may be observed while moving through branches, and in swimming reptiles such as sea turtles, gait evaluation is assessed best through observation of limb movement and propulsive force while swimming, if possible [3,43]. In terrestrial or semiaquatic chelonians that tend to resist manipulation by retreating into their shells, examination may be aided by placing the animal on an elevated platform, such as a small box or flowerpot, leaving the limbs in an unsupported position. When the animal decides to move, movement and strength of the limbs, neck, and head can be assessed. Snakes can be examined by allowing them to move through the examiner's hands, which also allows assessment of strength and muscle tone. Limbed reptiles should be able to support their weight, lift themselves off the ground, and move forward in a coordinated manner. Reptiles may exhibit various different gaits, which may be normal for certain individual species [1,44]. For example, snakes may display several different locomotory patterns, such as lateral undulation, concertina, sidewinding, and rectilinear movements [1,25,45].

Ataxia may manifest as stumbling to one or both sides, or as limbs crossing the midline plane. This may be accompanied by abnormalities in head position, such as a head tilt or opisthotonus (stargazing). Dysmetria also may be noted, characterized by hypometria (movements falling short of the intended goal) or hypermetria (exaggerated movements overreaching the intended goal).

Weakness may manifest as dragging of one or more limbs, or difficulty in raising the head or standing. Most snakes are able to maintain a horizontal plane with the cranial third or so of their body when held elevated, and can move up a vertical surface such as the walls of an enclosure. Chelonians should be able to retract their limbs and heads or hold them in a horizontal or partially elevated position. Failure to do so may indicate weakness caused by muscle or nervous system disease (Fig. 1). Snakes with spinal lesions may be unable to move the musculature adjacent to the lesion, resulting in abnormal gaits [46,47].

Occasionally, reptile patients may move in circles, usually in one direction, and typically toward the side of their neurologic lesion. Compulsive movement in a wide arc is usually indicative of cerebral (ie, telencephalic) disease, while moving in smaller, tighter circles, often accompanied by ataxia or rolling to one side is characteristic of vestibular dysfunction. Aquatic reptiles with neurologic disease may swim in circles, although other disease conditions affecting buoyancy (eg, pneumonia, free coelomic air, gastric bloat) can lead to similar behavior [14,15,20,48] and must be ruled out.

Cranial nerve examination

As in mammals, cranial nerve (CN) examination in reptiles can be useful in localizing lesions to regions of the brain or peripheral cranial nerves. There is considerable anatomic variation that must be kept in mind when performing these tests, however. Some reptiles may lack certain nerves or anatomical structures normally present in mammals (eg, eyelids), making certain tests impossible to perform. Conversely, in some cases, reptiles

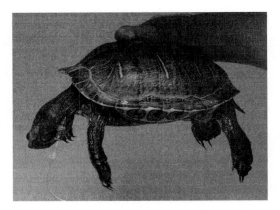

Fig. 1. Flaccid paralysis in a red-eared slider. This turtle was unable to raise the head and limbs, and withdrawal reflexes were absent. Electrodiagnostic evaluation confirmed diffuse lower motor neuron disease, and blood lead levels were elevated markedly.

may possess additional structures, such as infrared receptors in crotalids (pit vipers) and boid snakes [49]. The 12 cranial nerves normally described and evaluated in mammals (CN I to XII) are more or less present in reptiles, with some modifications (Table 1).

Table 1
The cranial nerves and their function

Number	Name	Innervation	Function(s)
VN	Vomeronasal	Vomeronasal organ	Chemosensation
I	Olfactory	Nasal epithelium	Olfaction
II	Optic	Retina	Vision
III	Oculomotor	Dorsal, ventral, and medial rectus muscles; ventral oblique muscle; iris	Movement of globe, pupil constriction
IV	Trochlear	Dorsal oblique muscle	Rotation of globe
V	Trigeminal	Sensory receptors on face and cornea, muscles of mastication, depressor palpebrae muscle	Sensation to face and cornea, jaw closure, lowers lower eyelid
VI	Abducens	Lateral rectus and retractor bulbi muscles	Movement of globe laterally, globe retraction
VII	Facial	Eyelid musculature, some jaw musculature, taste receptors on rostral tongue	Eyelid closure, opening jaw, taste to rostral tongue
VIII	Vestibulocochlear (Statoacoustic)	Semicircular canals, utricle, saccule, cochlea	Equilibrium, hearing
IX	Glossopharyngeal	Taste receptors on caudal tongue and pharynx, pharyngeal musculature	Taste to caudal tongue and pharynx, swallowing
X	Vagus	Most visceral organs, pharyngeal, esophageal, and laryngeal musculature	Parasympathetic functions of visceral organs, taste, swallowing, laryngeal function
XI[a]	Spinal accessory	Neck and shoulder musculature	Neck and shoulder movement
XII	Hypoglossal	Tongue musculature	Movement of tongue

The Cranial Nerves and their Function.
[a] Absent in snakes and some lizards.

Olfaction is an important sense for many reptiles [50,51]. Olfactory information is relayed to the brain by CN I. In addition, most reptiles have a vomeronasal organ, which is an accessory chemosensory apparatus that is innervated by the vomeronasal nerve. Tongue flicking in snakes and some lizards brings chemosensory information in contact with the vomeronasal organ, located just above the roof of the mouth. These nerves rarely are evaluated in clinical patients. Questioning the owner or caretaker about the animal's willingness to eat, however, may provide clues to dysfunction. Lesions also may result in ineffective sensing of pheromones and altered courtship behavior. Testing olfaction directly with the use of strong-smelling substances is also possible, although care should be taken with interpreting responses to noxious stimuli (eg, alcohol), as these also may stimulate the receptors in the nasal mucosa innervated by the trigeminal nerve.

Vision is assessed initially while observing the animal navigate in its environment. Obstacles may be placed in the animal's path or held in its field of view to observe a behavioral response. A menace response assesses the ability to see a threatening gesture and to close the eyelids in response. This can be performed with the hand or a held object such as a cotton swab. Note that snakes, amphisbaenians, and some lizards (eg, geckos) do not have eyelids and obviously cannot show this response. These tests assess ocular structures (eg, retina), CN II, the optic chiasm and tracts, the cerebral cortex, and in the case of the menace response, the cerebellum.

Size and appearance of the pupils should be noted, and anisocoria can be seen with some diseases [52,53]. The pupillary light reflex (PLR) in mammals is elicited by shining a bright light into one eye and looking for pupillary constriction of that eye (direct PLR) and of the contralateral eye (indirect PLR). It assesses CN II (senses the light) and CN III (constricts the pupil). Note that the reptilian iris is composed of skeletal muscle [11,25,54], and that the pupil may escape from constriction voluntarily while the light is still on. An initial constriction, however, usually is seen in the eye that the light is shone into (ie, direct response). The indirect PLR is difficult to appreciate in reptiles.

Cranial nerve III also innervates four of the six extraocular muscles. As a result, dysfunction of CN III may result in mydriasis or ventrolateral strabismus. Cranial nerve IV innervates the dorsal oblique muscle, which partly rotates the globe, while CN VI innervates the lateral rectus and retractor bulbi muscles. Dysfunction of the former may result in a rotational strabismus, which may be difficult to appreciate in animals with a round pupil without retinal examination. Lesions of CN VI may manifest as a medial strabismus. Note that true chameleons normally can move their eyes independently, which should not be mistaken for strabismus.

The trigeminal nerve (CN V) is responsible for sensation to the face and head and innervation of the muscles of mastication. As in mammals, it is comprised of three branches: the ophthalmic, maxillary, and mandibular. In some reptiles (pit vipers and boid snakes), CN V is also responsible for innervating the heat-sensing infrared receptors [22]. Although not reported to the author's knowledge, CN V dysfunction in these species in theory may lead to difficulty in food capture, which might be perceived as inappetence. Palpebral reflexes usually can be elicited in species with eyelids, making it possible to evaluate CN V (sensation) and CN VII (motor). This test is performed best with a cotton swab, especially in smaller species. In most species, the upper eyelid has little mobility, and the lower lid moves dorsally to cover the eye [25]. Facial sensation also can be evaluated by gentle pricking with a small needle or in some cases by insertion of a blunt-tipped object into the nostrils and looking for a behavioral response. The presence of a dropped jaw or masticatory muscle atrophy may indicate dysfunction of the mandibular branch. Therefore, CN V dysfunction may result in difficulty in prehension or chewing of food. Note that in many lizards and in snakes, the maxilla also moves independently of the mandible, which aids in feeding on large prey. The corneal reflex may be performed by lightly touching the cornea with a moistened cotton swab or wisp of cotton material, which results in closing of the eyelids and globe retraction. This reflex assesses CN V (sensation), CN VI (globe retraction), and CN VII (eyelid closure).

The facial nerve (CN VII) innervates the muscles of facial expression (or head musculature other than the muscles of mastication). It is assessed with the palpebral response described previously, and by observing facial symmetry. This nerve can be difficult to assess in reptiles because of a lack of moveable lips and pinnae (and eyelids in some species). Snakes and many species of lizards have developed cranial kinesis, defined as the ability to move the upper and lower jaw, facilitating capture and swallowing of prey. Cranial nerve VII innervates the musculature responsible for opening the jaw, and dysfunction might manifest as difficulty in feeding. The sensory portion of CN VII is responsible for taste sensation in the cranial two thirds of the tongue. It is possible to assess this with the application of a bitter substance (eg, atropine) placed on a cotton swab and touched to the side of the tongue, which results in an adverse response and avoidance behavior.

The vestibulocochlear (statoacoustic) nerve (CN VIII) is responsible for both hearing and the sense of equilibrium or balance. Hearing can be difficult to assess in reptiles, and even the ability to hear has been questioned for some species, as they lack external ear canals, tympanic membranes, and in some cases, middle ear structures. Experimental studies have shown, however, that most species are able to perceive airborne stimuli, although sounds are best heard at lower frequencies (see brainstem auditory evoked response testing section). Some animals will respond to a loud noise, although assessing each ear independently is extremely difficult.

The vestibular portion of CN VIII is assessed by observing the gait and position of the head and eyes. Reptiles with vestibular lesions may show a head tilt (usually to the side of the lesion) [48,55], ataxia, and spontaneous nystagmus [3]. As in birds with nystagmus, the whole head may move with fast and slow phases in conjunction with the eyes. The eyes also should be evaluated for the presence of normal physiologic nystagmus and for evidence of positional nystagmus or strabismus, often characterized as a ventral strabismus with head elevation on the side of the lesion. The tympanic membranes should be evaluated for swelling associated with aural abscessation, a common condition in chelonians [26].

The glossopharyngeal (CN IX) and vagus (CN X) nerves typically are evaluated together, but to a limited extent. They are responsible for the pharyngeal and esophageal musculature, and dysfunction may result in dysphagia or regurgitation. These nerves are also responsible for taste receptors on the caudal tongue and pharynx. Additional autonomic functions include innervation of baroreceptors (CN IX) and most of the viscera (CN X). These activities are difficult to assess, but signs of dysfunction may be seen with other parts of the physical examination, such as the assessment of heart rate or gastrointestinal (GI) function.

Cranial nerve XI is the spinal accessory nerve, and it innervates muscles of the neck and shoulder (sternocleidohyoideus, trapezius) and the larynx. There is some confusion over the identification of this nerve in different species, as it may be composed of spinal nerve rootlets and the caudal rootlets of CN X [1,56]. It is apparently absent in snakes and some lizards [1,56,57]. In limbed reptiles, CN XI function may be assessed by observation and palpation of the associated musculature.

The hypoglossal nerve (CN XII) innervates the tongue musculature, and can be assessed by watching for normal tongue movement, position, tone, and symmetry. Regular tongue flicking should be noted in snakes (and some lizard species) during the examination. Opening of the mouth to assess this and other cranial nerves can be facilitated with the use of a plastic card, rubber spatula, or in some heavy-jawed species, an avian beak speculum. Some lizards will open their mouth in response to tapping on the nose or with gentle traction on the dewlap.

Posture and postural reactions

The position of the head and neck should be noted. Most reptiles are able to lift and move their head freely. Abnormalities of head position may include head tilts (ie, off the horizontal axis) [55], head turns (ie, off the vertical axis), or opisthotonus (stargazing or dorsal flexion of the head and neck) [52]. A behavioral stargazing has been described in captive boid snakes, which may be related to feeding practices, but these animals are able to maintain normal head posture most of the time [42]. Ventral flexion and inability to lift the head may be related to generalized weakness due to a variety of causes (see Fig. 1). Abnormal head movements include tremors and seizure activity [55]. Head bobbing while breathing has been associated with respiratory infections in tortoises and box turtles, and might be confused with neurologic dysfunction [20]. Abnormal spinal curvature, including kyphosis, lordosis, or scoliosis may be seen, caused by congenital malformations or ankylosis from acquired conditions [46]. Some animals may lay in lateral or dorsal recumbency. Uneven floating in aquatic turtles may be a result of conditions affecting buoyancy (see gait examination previously).

The assessment of postural reactions in dogs and cats often consists of tests such as hopping, hemiwalking or hemistanding, wheelbarrowing, limb-placing responses, and the assessment of conscious proprioception by turning the paw over so that the dorsal surface comes in contact with the ground. Some of these tests can be adapted for the evaluation of the limbed reptiles. The utility of turning feet over is somewhat limited in this group of animals, but may be accomplished in some lizards. Assessment of responses to hopping, wheelbarrowing, and placing responses (by bringing a limb up to the edge of a table) may provide more useful information. Postural sense also may be assessed partly by having an animal stand on a sheet of paper (or similar moveable surface) and then slowly moving the paper laterally, observing for return of the limb to a normal position.

Spinal reflexes

Spinal cord reflexes in mammals are thought to occur segmentally; that is, they require afferent and efferent peripheral nerves, and a connection within the spinal cord at a certain level, without the need for ascending or descending control. A lesion above or below this spinal cord level will not interfere with the function of the reflex, although lesions at a higher (ie, rostral) level may result in a loss of descending inhibition and an exaggerated response. The pathways are not documented as well in reptiles, but anatomical studies suggest that spinal reflexes should function segmentally [1,58].

The evaluation of segmental spinal reflexes in dogs and cats usually includes myotatic reflexes (such as the patellar reflex), withdrawal reflexes (elicited after squeezing on a digit), and the anal reflex (constriction of the anal sphincter after stimulation). Many of the myotatic reflexes are unreliable, even in dogs and cats, and these should be interpreted with caution in reptilian patients, if attempted [3]. Withdrawal reflexes can be elicited reliably from most legged reptiles, after squeezing on a digit or pricking the plantar surface of the limb with a sharp object. A cloacal reflex, similar to the anal reflex in mammals, also can often be elicited by stimulation of the cloaca with a cotton swab, hemostat, or similar instrument. Contraction of the cloacal musculature is the normal response. In some animals, the tail also may move ventrally as part of this reflex, and in turtles, the pelvic limbs normally will come together in a clasp response [3,4]. Loss of cloacal tone has been reported for spinal cord injuries presumably occurring above the spinal cord level expected for cloacal innervation, and the segmental nature of the cloacal reflex remains undocumented [4,5,22]. Crossed extensor reflexes, when seen in mammals, are interpreted as an exaggerated response, indicating an upper motor neuron lesion and a loss of descending inhibition.

Although some authors state that crossed extensor reflexes are seen in reptiles normally, this has not been reported by others [3], and it is not typical of normal animals in this author's experience.

Studies performed in experimental animals illustrate the capacity of the reptilian spinal cord to generate complex movements without supraspinal input. For example, a scratch reflex is seen in turtles with complete spinal cord transection [1,59,60]. Cutaneous stimulation below the level of the lesion elicits movement of a pelvic limb, which reaches forward to touch the stimulated site with a scratching motion. This movement is generated entirely within the spinal cord by central pattern generators, and is not voluntary, demonstrating the tremendous autonomy of the reptilian spinal cord [59]. Such systems may prove beneficial for recovery from severe spinal cord injury (see prognosis section).

Other responses and reflexes

A panniculus reflex may be elicited by gently pricking the skin on either side of the spine with a needle and observing a twitch of the skin and underlying musculature, as in mammals [4,5,12]. This is obviously impossible in chelonian species. It usually is lost caudal to the level of a spinal cord lesion.

Most reptiles are able to rapidly return to a normal upright posture after being placed in dorsal recumbency (the so-called righting reflex), and failure to do so may indicate underlying neurologic disease. Whereas lizards and chelonians (sea turtles also) use their necks and limbs in an attempt to right themselves, snakes rapidly turn their heads over, followed by the rest of the body. This test can be useful in identifying the level of a spinal cord lesion in snakes, as the part of the body caudal to the lesion may remain upturned [4]. Note that some lizards and crocodilians may enter a trance-like state when placed in dorsal recumbency with stroking of their abdomen; this response is seen in normal animals and will inhibit the righting reflex.

Assessment of pain, muscle size, and tone

Spinal palpation may reveal areas of pain associated with lesions of the spine, muscle, or nerve root. Lesions affecting the spine or skull can be palpated or visualized in some cases (Fig. 2). They may include kyphosis, lordosis, scoliosis, or ankylosis associated with congenital malformations, osteomyelitis, osteoarthritis, osteoarthrosis, or instability related to pathologic or traumatic fractures [4,46,47]. Muscles of the trunk and limbs can be palpated for evidence of pain, loss of tone, or atrophy associated with either focal or generalized lesions. In chelonians with paraparesis, palpation of the abdomen for retained eggs, soft tissue masses, impactions, or other space-occupying lesions is prudent, as these may put pressure on the sciatic nerves in the enclosed area within the shell [14].

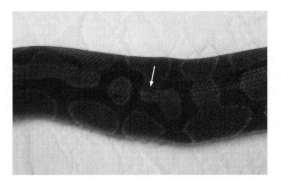

Fig. 2. Visual identification of a traumatic spinal lesion in a snake (*arrow*).

Pain sensation in veterinary medicine traditionally has been separated into superficial and deep pain perception [6,7]. Superficial sensation is assessed by pinching of the skin with hemostats or pricking the skin with a small needle. Loss of sensation in certain dermatomes over the head, trunk, or limbs helps to localize lesions to certain regions of the central or peripheral nervous systems. This has been described in reptilian patients [3].

More important in many situations is the assessment of so-called deep pain. This is assessed by exerting firm pressure on the periosteum by squeezing over the bone of a digit or tail vertebrae with hemostats, pliers, or a similar instrument. Although a withdrawal reflex often is elicited, the appropriate response for pain sensation is cerebral recognition of the stimulus, manifested as turning of the head toward the examiner, or attempts to escape or bite. It is used primarily as a prognostic indicator for animals with spinal cord injury, as the pathways for deep pain are almost always the last to lose function with this type of lesion, indicating a severe injury (see prognosis section).

Localization of lesions within the nervous system

Lesion localization in reptiles uses the same principles as in mammals, and it is modified as necessary because of differences in anatomy. For example, snakes may have hundreds of vertebrae with corresponding spinal cord segments that generally are not classified into cervical, thoracic, or lumbar segments, but are instead numbered sequentially from head to tail (or pre- and postcloacal). Chelonians have 18 precloacal vertebrae (eight cervical and 10 thoracic/dorsal), while lizards and crocodilians have variable numbers of thoracic and lumbar vertebrae. Limbed species have enlargements of the spinal cord corresponding to the brachial and lumbar intumescences [1]. Localization of a neurologic lesion may be accomplished by performing the tests described previously, and then combining this with an appropriate history from the owner or caretaker to fit the lesion into one of several categories described in Box 1.

Box 1. Categories of neurologic lesions

Prosencephalon (telencephalon and diencephalon; forebrain): evidence of seizures, altered mentation, behavioral changes, visual or olfactory deficits, contralateral limb paresis or postural reaction deficits

Mesencephalon (midbrain): altered mentation, contralateral or ipsilateral limb paresis or postural reaction deficits, CN III or IV dysfunction

Rhombencephalon (metencephalon and myelencephalon; pons and medulla oblongata): altered mentation, ipsilateral limb paresis or postural reaction deficits, CN V-XII dysfunction

Cerebellum (metencephalon, in part): ataxia, intention tremors, dysmetria, possible vestibular dysfunction (head tilt, nystagmus)

Cervical spinal cord: paresis and ataxia in all four limbs (or trunk caudal to lesion), normal spinal reflexes, pain on spine, or muscle palpation

Spinal cord at the level of the brachial intumescence: paresis and ataxia in all four limbs (or trunk caudal to lesion), reduced to absent thoracic limb withdrawal reflexes, pain on spine or muscle palpation

Spinal cord between the brachial and lumbar intumescences: paresis and ataxia in pelvic limbs (or trunk caudal to lesion), normal segmental spinal reflexes, pain on spine or muscle palpation; panniculus and/or righting reflex may be useful in further defining level of lesion

Spinal cord at the level of the lumbar intumescence: paresis and ataxia in pelvic limbs (or trunk caudal to lesion), reduced to absent pelvic limb withdrawal reflexes, cloacal reflex and/or clasp reflex, pain on spine or muscle palpation

Spinal cord caudal to the lumbar intumescence: weak, paralyzed, and/or flaccid tail, pain on spine or muscle palpation

Multifocal: lesions affecting multiple areas of the CNS ± peripheral nervous system (PNS), not explainable by a lesion in a single anatomic location

PNS: weakness or ataxia in all four limbs, reduced to absent spinal reflexes in all four limbs, ± cranial nerve dysfunction

Neuromuscular junction: generalized weakness (continuous or episodic); segmental spinal reflexes may be normal (with episodic diseases), reduced or absent (with continuous conditions), ± cranial nerve dysfunction

Muscle: generalized weakness, normal spinal reflexes, muscle pain, muscle atrophy

Prognosis

The prognosis for survival or return to function obviously depends on the disease process. For spinal cord injury in mammals, the prognosis for return to function correlates to a certain degree with the presence or absence of deep pain sensation, indicating a functionally incomplete or complete injury respectively. Although well-documented in traditional small animal medicine, this correlation has not been established in reptiles. In fact, some studies have determined that reptiles may recover locomotory function after experimental spinal cord hemisection [61] or transection [62], suggesting that the prognosis for reptiles with severe spinal cord injury is better than it is in mammals [2,12]. This may be related to the role of central pattern generators within the spinal cord, and greater autonomy of these structures, so that they may function without higher brainstem or cortical input [63].

These studies, however, did not comment on GI or urinary tract function, which often complicates recovery from spinal cord injury in reptiles, and must be taken into consideration. In general, reptiles may show dramatic recoveries from various injuries to the nervous system. Therefore, giving them a chance to recover can be rewarding in many cases.

Clinical pathology

Blood tests

Blood tests can be very useful in identifying diseases affecting the nervous system, and collection and analysis of blood has been described well in reptiles [48,64]. A complete blood count may show a leukocytosis associated with infectious disease [4,12,52] or evidence of lymphoid neoplasia or leukemia, which may affect the nervous system [12,65,66]. Anemia with evidence of a regenerative erythrocytic response and basophilic stippling may be seen with lead intoxication.

Serum biochemical evaluation may disclose several abnormalities related to neurologic dysfunction. Muscle tremors, fasciculations, and seizures may be caused by hypocalcemia, which is seen most often in green iguanas [12,20,67]. Hypoglycemia leading to neurologic signs (mydriasis, altered mentation, opisthotonus) has been described in crocodilians [2,4,68]. Hyponatremia and hypernatremia can cause altered mentation and seizures in mammals and theoretically may lead to similar signs in reptilian patients. Hepatic and renal encephalopathy have been described in reptiles [4,9,22,48,69] and may have corresponding abnormalities on biochemical evaluation. Cholesterol may be elevated in patients with xanthomas (cholesterol granulomas), which can occur in the brain [4,70,71]. Elevations of creatine kinase may be seen with vitamin E or selenium deficiency [40] or other muscle diseases.

Serum bile acid evaluation has been described in reptiles [72,73], and may be useful to identify liver dysfunction associated with hepatic encephalopathy. Lead intoxication may be confirmed with blood lead levels [29,64,74], and assays for other toxins may be useful also. A reduced serum cholinesterase level suggests organophosphate intoxication.

Infectious disease tests

Infectious diseases are important causes of neurologic disease in reptiles, and these may include bacterial [10,22,47,75,76], mycoplasmal [77,78], viral [4,55,79–91] or suspected viral [10,52,92–94], fungal [53,95–98], protozoal [4,14,22,99–101], and parasitic [3,4,102,103] etiologies. Bacterial and fungal cultures can be obtained from blood, body fluids, or tissue as in other species [26,46,47,64,76,95,96,104,105]. Serological tests for some diseases associated with CNS disease are available [90], including chelonian herpes virus [64,87], ophidian paramyxovirus [4,64,82,84], ophidian reovirus [64], and West Nile virus [81,106]. Much effort has been devoted to developing a test for inclusion body disease, which is seen primarily in boid snakes, and is suspected to be caused by a retrovirus [52,107,108]. Other antemortem diagnostic techniques available for infectious diseases include cytology, histology and immunohistochemistry, virus isolation, and polymerase chain reaction (PCR) [52,55,64,77,82,87,89,90,109–112].

Cerebrospinal fluid analysis

In mammals, three layers of meninges surround the CNS (the pia, arachnoid, and dura maters), and cerebrospinal fluid (CSF) flows caudally from the ventricular system of the brain into the subarachnoid space surrounding the brain and spinal cord. Reptiles possess only two meningeal layers (an outer dura and an inner leptomeninx), and it has been stated that CSF collection is impossible in these animals, as there is no subarachnoid space [113]. CSF, however, is produced by the choroid plexus within the ventricular system, and flows caudally in a subdural space in reptiles. This CSF can be obtained for analysis [22,48,64,114–117], although collection is more challenging than it is for most mammalian species [53,96,104,118].

As in mammals, collection of CSF can be attempted at two main locations: the atlanto–occipital (AO) space and in the lumbar region. Collection at the latter location is particularly challenging, and although the spinal cord typically ends more caudally than it does in mammals [1,57,64,113], obtaining CSF in amounts suitable for analysis can be very difficult. For collection at the AO space, reptilian patients may be placed in either ventral or lateral recumbency, and they typically are anesthetized, although this may not be required in all cases with adequate physical restraint. The animal's head should be held in a ventrally flexed position (Fig. 3). Landmarks will vary by species but are somewhat intuitive for those accustomed to performing this procedure in mammalian species. The caudal edge of the skull is palpated, and the needle entry point is a short distance behind

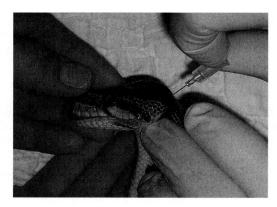

Fig. 3. Cerebrospinal fluid collection in a snake. An assistant holds the animal's head steady in a ventroflexed position. The needle is passed between the occipital bones of the skull and the first cervical vertebrae. A spinal needle may be used, although in small patients, a regular needle is easier, as it allows better visualization of cerebrospinal fluid (CSF) flow and requires less manipulation, reducing the likelihood of iatrogenic hemorrhage and blood contamination.

this point, cranial to the atlas, if this structure can be palpated. A spinal needle is preferred, although a regular hypodermic needle can be used for collection in smaller patients.

The main difficulty with obtaining CSF, in the author's experience, is the lack of spontaneous flow in smaller patients, even when the needle is in the correct position. Although some have suggested aspiration with a syringe to obtain greater quantities [22,64,116,119], this must be performed with caution, as blood contamination and damage to the CNS tissue is possible. Even when no visible flow is observed, enough CSF may move through capillary action up the needle to facilitate cytologic evaluation (Fig. 4). In some species (eg, chelonians, crocodilians), a blood sinus may be present overlying the dura and subdural space [118], and a spinal needle with stylet is required to traverse this sinus to obtain CSF. Ultrasound also may be used to guide the needle into the correct location (D Heard, BVMS, personal communication, 2006). In large species such as the American alligator, CSF will flow freely up the needle with the animal in ventral recumbency, and can be collected as it flows over the edge of the needle hub with a syringe or sample tube.

Reports of CSF analysis in reptiles are extremely limited. A study evaluating CSF from clinically normal American alligators showed cell counts similar to mammalian CSF, but markedly elevated protein levels [120]. Ideally, these tests, and cytologic evaluation, should be performed as soon as possible after sample collection to avoid degradation of the cells. Meningo-encephalitis and meningomyelitis generally result in increases in the white cell count and protein level of the CSF. In the absence of normal values for most reptilian species, mammalian values can be used as a guideline. Infectious organisms may be seen in some cases on cytologic evaluation [10,22], and might be facilitated by special staining (eg, for acid-fast

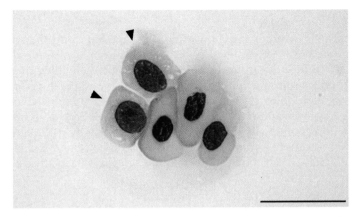

Fig. 4. Cytologic evaluation of a CSF sample obtained from the atlanto–occipital space in a bearded dragon. This sample showed mild blood contamination, as evidenced by the erythrocytes (cells on lower right) next to the small mononuclear cells (*arrowheads*). A limited amount of CSF could be obtained from this patient, limiting examination to cytology. Excessive numbers of leukocytes present on a non-concentrated smear, however, suggested meningoencephalitis. Scale bar = 20 μm.

organisms) [4,22]. Positive culture and PCR analysis of CSF for mycoplasma also have been described [114,121]. Hematologic malignancies are relatively common in reptiles, and may involve the nervous system [65,122,123]. Although not reported to the author's knowledge, it is possible that neoplastic cells might be visualized within the CSF of animals with cancers such as lymphoma.

Diagnostic imaging

Radiography

Radiographic techniques to examine the skull and spine of reptiles are relatively easy to perform and have been documented by other authors [10,124–133]. The reader is referred to these reports for details regarding positioning, technique, and other technical aspects of this modality. Radiography can be useful to visualize spinal lesions resulting from trauma [5,129,134,135], congenital malformations [22,33,127], nutritional or renal secondary hyperparathyroidism (ie, metabolic bone disease) [129,131], osteomyelitis [10,47,76,129], proliferative osteoarthritis [22,46,127], and neoplasia [136]. Skull lesions identified may include traumatic fractures, bony lysis associated with aural abscessation, or neoplasia [26]. Female chelonians may develop paraparesis or paraplegia because of retention of eggs or other space-occupying masses within the caudal abdomen, which may be visualized radiographically [5,12,14]. Gout may cause crystal formation within the articular joints of the spine or the CNS itself, and this might be identified with radiography in some cases [4].

Myelography

Myelography requires injection of contrast medium into the space normally occupied by CSF, to identify compressive lesions affecting the spinal cord. As a result, it is subject to many of the same difficulties encountered with CSF collection and has been considered very difficult or impossible to perform in reptiles [127]. Myelography has been reported in lizards [129,137], however, and is seemingly feasible in other reptile species. Compressive lesions potentially identifiable with myelography include traumatic fractures or luxations, granulomas or soft tissue swelling associated with infectious disease, congenital malformations, and neoplastic disease.

Ultrasonography

Ultrasonography of the nervous system is challenging in any vertebrate species because of the encasement of the entire CNS within a protective bony skull and spine. Visualization of the CNS in mammals usually is accomplished through persistent foraminae (eg, bregmatic fontanelle in hydrocephalic dogs), although normal anatomic acoustic windows also can be used [138]. The author is not aware of any reports of ultrasound to evaluate the reptilian nervous system. The brain of avian patients, however, often can be imaged through the skull with transducers of appropriate frequency, and this also might be possible in some smaller, thin-skulled reptilian patients.

Nuclear scintigraphy

The use of nuclear scintigraphy has been described infrequently in reptiles and other exotic species [127,129,133,139,140]. This technique uses radioactive tracers, which concentrate in areas of active bone remodeling (or other tissues of interest), and are then visualized subsequently with an appropriate detection device (eg, gamma camera). The main disadvantages of these techniques are the low resolution of the images obtained, low specificity, and the difficulties associated with the handling of radioactive materials and waste. Lesions of the skull and spine, such as osteomyelitis, traumatic lesions, or vertebral neoplasia, potentially may be identified with this modality [140], and its use to identify brain tumors has been described [129].

CT

The use of advanced, cross-sectional imaging techniques has revolutionized human, and subsequently veterinary, medicine. CT uses x-ray beams passed through the patient and captured as a series of transverse slices, to generate a gray-scale image of the area in question. Although images can be captured only in a single plane without repositioning of the patient, the images can be reconstructed digitally in multiple planes with appropriate computer software. As with conventional radiography, CT displays bone as bright white, air as black, and soft tissue structures as various shades of gray. Images can be manipulated digitally, or windowed to highlight different tissues of interest.

CT can be very useful in identifying lesions affecting the nervous system of reptile patients. Numerous reports describing CT of reptiles are available [125,127,130,133,140–150]. CT is more sensitive than conventional radiography, and it may allow visualization of lesions not detected with plain radiographs, particularly in chelonians, where superimposed shell structures may complicate assessment [141–143,146,151]. It is most valuable in identifying bony lesions affecting the vertebrae and skull. With the addition of intravenous contrast material (eg, iohexol), however, enhancement of lesions within the CNS such as neoplasia and meningoencephalitis may be appreciated. Acute hemorrhage usually is visualized well with CT. Bony lesions easily identified on CT include skull or vertebral fractures, otitis media-interna, osteomyelitis, and neoplasia [130,133,140,142,145,149]. The thoracic (dorsal) spinal canal (ie, portion attached to the carapace) in chelonians appears remarkably small in normal individuals, and should not be considered mistakenly as a diseased segment causing spinal cord compression (Fig. 5).

MRI

Similar to CT, MRI is a method of cross-sectional imaging that has revolutionized the practice of medicine. MRI, however, is superior to CT in numerous ways, including a lack of ionizing radiation, the ability to perform true (ie, nonreconstructed) imaging in multiple planes, and vastly superior detail of soft tissue structures, including nervous tissue within the CNS and PNS. MRI uses an entirely different technology than CT and relies

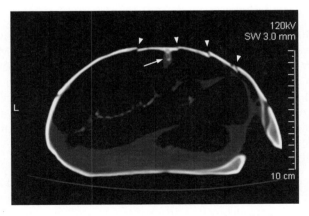

Fig. 5. Computed tomography image of a tortoise presented after vehicular trauma. The spinal canal of turtles and tortoises is remarkably narrow in the thoracic (dorsal) region of normal individuals, and is unaffected by the trauma in this animal (*arrow*). Note multiple fractures of the carapace, however (*arrowheads*).

on strong magnetic fields and radiofrequency pulses to produce images that highlight differences in water content between various tissues. Disadvantages of this imaging modality typically include the need for general anesthesia and contraindications associated with bringing patients with metallic (magnetic) implants into the imaging suite. The main purpose for anesthesia, however, is to prevent movement and subsequent motion artifact, and many patients, particularly chelonians, may be imaged without chemical restraint, or with sedation alone [148,152].

Although there are few available reports of MRI in reptiles [10,125,127,133,146–148,150,152–155], this modality can be extremely useful in visualizing the nervous system in these patients. Various conditions affecting the nervous system likely would be visualized well with MRI or CT, including cholesterol granulomas [70,71,156], abscesses [26], fungal granulomas, meningoencephalitis or meningomyelitis [53,55,87,94,96], vertebral osteomyelitis [47,95], hydrocephalus [4], and neoplastic disease [157,158].

Tumors of the CNS and PNS rarely have been reported in reptiles [4,123,156,157,159–166], and reviews of neoplastic disease in these animals infrequently report nervous system involvement [158,161,167–174]. Although this may be related to a relative paucity of these tumors compared with mammalian species, neurologic signs are often attributed to systemic illness, and the nervous system is less likely to be examined at necropsy. Thus, these tumors may be more common than has been appreciated, and advanced diagnostic imaging, particularly CT and MRI, provides the best noninvasive way to detect these lesions. In addition, tumors invading nervous tissue from adjacent areas [158,175–177] are appreciated best by these modalities.

Electrodiagnostic techniques

Electrodiagnostic techniques used for the evaluation of neurologic disease in veterinary patients have included electromyography (EMG), motor and sensory nerve conduction velocity, F wave evaluation, repetitive nerve stimulation, spinal cord evoked potentials (SEP), and electroencephalography (EEG). Many of these techniques can be applied to unconventional species. A review of clinical electrodiagnostic testing in exotic animals has been published [178], although the evaluation of reptiles was not described.

Electromyography

EMG frequently is performed by veterinary neurologists, and it evaluates the intrinsic electrical activity of muscle. It is performed by inserting active and recording electrodes (often incorporated into the same needle) into a muscle belly, which produces waveforms that can be evaluated visually and acoustically [179–181]. Insertion of the needle produces a short burst of activity, known as the insertional potential. Although contracting muscles produce regular electrical activity, the EMG of a normal muscle at rest should be electrically silent. In veterinary patients, this procedure typically is performed under general anesthesia to prevent unwanted muscle contraction. Denervation of muscle or intrinsic disease of the muscle itself produces abnormal potentials that have characteristic waveforms and sounds. These include fibrillation potentials (which sound like frying eggs or bacon), positive sharp waves (which make a popping sound or sound like a revving engine), and complex repetitive discharges (which sound like a dive-bombing airplane).

EMG is performed easily in most reptilian species, and the interpretation is identical to mammalian patients. The needle often needs to be directed between dermal scutes or scales, but the muscle underneath typically is accessed without difficulty (Fig. 6). Generalized abnormal potentials may be observed with polyneuropathies (axonal disease) or diffuse muscle disease (Fig. 7). The EMG cannot distinguish reliably between these two disease processes, and further electrodiagnostic testing with or without muscle and/or nerve biopsy usually is required. Focal disease of a single nerve, group of nerves, or focal muscle group also can be detected with this technique.

Motor nerve conduction velocity

This test involves stimulation of a selected nerve at two or more points, with recording of a resulting compound muscle action potential (CMAP) within a muscle innervated by the nerve [180,182]. The recording needle is identical to the needles used for EMG. The time taken for the CMAP to be generated after stimulation (latency) is recorded for each stimulation point. If the distance between the stimulation points is measured, a velocity

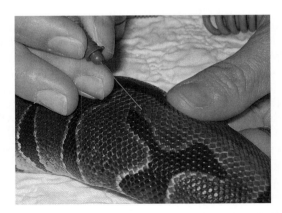

Fig. 6. Electromyography in a snake. All of the axial musculature is available for examination with this modality, using techniques identical to those used for mammalian species. Note the angle of the recording needle electrode, which is directed between scales to access the underlying musculature.

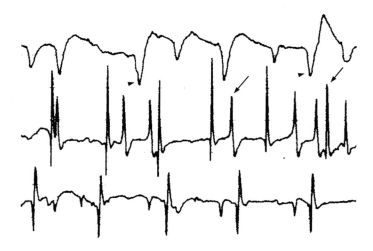

Fig. 7. Electromyographic tracings from the snake pictured in Fig. 6. The lines represent three separate (ie, noncontinuous) captured traces from the examination. Fibrillation potentials (*arrows*) and positive sharp waves (*arrowheads*) were found focally in this snake, adjacent to a traumatic spinal lesion. The bottom tracing shows a regularly repeating waveform, consistent with nonpathologic motor unit action potentials. Note that, by convention, a positive deflection is downwards in an electromyogram (EMG) record.

of conduction along this nerve can be calculated. The CMAP also can be evaluated for its amplitude, duration, and overall appearance of the wave-form [180,182]. Even more so than in mammals, it is important that this test be performed while the animal is at appropriate body temperatures, as low temperatures will reduce nerve conduction velocity [4,183].

Demyelinating peripheral nerve disease can result in reduced motor nerve conduction velocity, and this may increase the overall CMAP latency or lead to a polyphasic waveform. Axonal disease or muscle disease may result in a reduction of the CMAP amplitude. Thus, this test, together with EMG, is helpful in differentiating neuropathic from myopathic disease processes. In patients with trauma, this test also can be useful to document anatomical or functional transection of a nerve (as an all-or-none CMAP response to stimulation).

Motor nerve conduction velocity can be performed on reptile patients, albeit with some limitations. Obviously, the anatomy and course of the nerve to be evaluated must be known. In mammals, this test typically is per-formed on appendicular nerves, although techniques for evaluating the CMAP of other nerves, such as the trigeminal, facial, and recurrent laryn-geal nerves, have been described [184,185]. The accuracy of the velocity mea-surement depends on reliable measurement of the distance between the recording sites. Short distances make measurement more difficult and

exaggerate the inaccuracies associated with the procedure. As a result, a minimum recording distance of 10 cm has been suggested for ideal results [186],
and the accuracy of results in smaller patients may be compromised. In addition, the anatomy of certain species may limit stimulation sites (eg, the
carapace of some chelonians). Finally, normal values for reptiles have not
been established. Despite these limitations, however, recordings can be obtained in reptilian patients, and they may help to guide clinical decisions
(Fig. 8). The author has performed motor nerve conduction velocity successfully on turtles (red-eared sliders, sea turtles), tortoises, and lizards.

F wave evaluation and repetitive nerve stimulation

F wave elicitation and repetitive nerve stimulation are specialized electrodiagnostic procedures used to evaluate specific segments of the motor unit
(ie, motor neuron cell body, axon, and neuromuscular junction). They are
performed with the same equipment used for nerve conduction velocity.
The F wave is a late potential produced by retrograde transmission of an
impulse from the site of stimulation, up the ventral nerve root to the motor
neuron cell body, and then subsequent anterograde transmission to the
recording site in the muscle. It is used to evaluate the ventral nerve root
and proximal nerve [186,187].

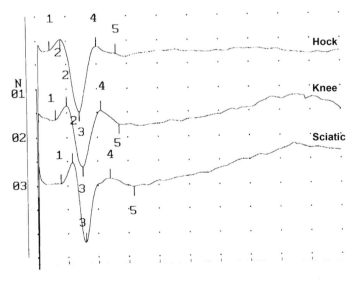

Fig. 8. Motor nerve conduction velocity measured in the left pelvic limb of the turtle pictured in
Fig. 1. The sciatic and tibial nerves were stimulated at three points, which elicited the compound
muscle action potentials shown (automatically labeled at points 1–5). After measuring the
distance between the stimulation points, the conduction velocity can be measured, which was
31.3 meters per second (m/s) proximally and 27.0 m/s distally in this case.

Repetitive nerve stimulation consists of rapid, repetitive stimulation of a nerve, while noting the amplitude of the CMAP produced with each stimulation. Diseases of the neuromuscular junction (eg, myasthenia gravis) may result in a decremental response, as transmission across the neuromuscular junction fails [186,188]. Both F wave evaluation and repetitive nerve stimulation can be performed in reptile patients, although no published reports are available to the author's knowledge (Fig. 9).

Brainstem auditory evoked response

The brainstem auditory evoked response (BAER) is a waveform produced after stimulation of the auditory nerve, and it corresponds to the transmission of impulses from this nerve, through associated nuclei and then ascending in the brainstem to higher brain centers [189]. In mammals, this response usually is recorded as a waveform with six to seven peaks [178,189–191]. It typically is elicited by playing a series of auditory clicks through headphones or tubal inserts into the ear canal, with recording, reference, and ground electrodes placed on the skin of the head [190,191]. A technique using bone conduction of sound also can be used [192,193]. This test can be useful to identify dysfunction of the auditory nerve itself, or disease processes affecting the brainstem along the pathway of transmission.

This test appears to be of limited value in reptilian patients, at least using stimulus parameters typically used for mammals. This may be because of the high frequency of the standard auditory click stimulus (which is a range centered at approximately 3200 Hz) [189,191]. In addition, anatomical variations make equipment placement difficult. Reptiles usually have a very short (lizards, crocodilians) or nonexistent (turtles, snakes) external ear canal [194], which precludes the placement of tubal inserts in most cases. Snakes lack both a tympanic membrane and a middle ear cavity [194], and traditionally have been considered deaf [195]. They do possess stapes (columella) and inner ear structures (a lagena or cochlea) however [194], and experimental studies indicate that they can perceive sound of airborne and seismic (ie, vibrational) origin [195]. Most reptiles appear to perceive sounds in low frequency ranges (approximately 150 to 600 Hz) [195]. As with other electrophysiologic testing in reptiles, auditory responses seem to be altered by temperature changes [196], and care should be taken to perform testing

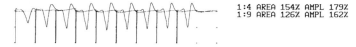

```
1:4 AREA 154% AMPL 179%
1:9 AREA 126% AMPL 162%
```

Fig. 9. Repetitive nerve stimulation of the tibial nerve, performed in the turtle shown in Fig. 1. The machine is set to compare the amplitude and area under the curve of the initial waveform with the fourth and ninth waveforms. A decremental response may indicate disease of the neuromuscular junction. In this case, an incremental response was seen, which was interpreted as normal.

at the animal's POTR. The author has not been successful in recording BAER from reptile species with typical mammalian stimulus parameters. It is possible, however, that employing lower frequencies, different intensities, or the use of a bone vibrator may enable these waveforms to be elicited in reptile patients. Other authors have been able to capture a BAER from reptiles with airborne sound [197], albeit under more invasive, experimental recording conditions, and responses from loggerhead sea turtles using a vibrational stimulus have been reported [198].

Spinal cord evoked response

The spinal cord evoked response (or somatosensory evoked potential) is a waveform elicited after stimulation of the nerve of a pelvic or thoracic limb and recorded from the spinal cord itself at a point rostral to the stimulation site [199,200]. The recording electrode is placed ideally on the dorsal surface of the dura mater, or alternatively, in contact with the dorsal lamina of a vertebra. This test may provide information regarding the speed of conduction of impulses in the spinal cord, and it has been used to detect areas of spinal cord injury [201]. In certain areas of the spinal cord corresponding to neuronal synapses, this technique can record a very large waveform (cord dorsum potential), which is a field (sink source) potential related to extracellular ion movements [186,199,200].

The author and others (SR Platt, unpublished data, 1998, [2]) have used this technique in an attempt to identify chelonian patients with functionally transected spinal cords (ie, complete spinal lesions). Trauma to the shell of tortoises and turtles frequently results in spinal cord trauma because of the intimate association of the vertebrae with the carapace. In theory, this technique may provide an assessment of the integrity of the spinal cord, and therefore, the possibility for recovery in these patients. The stimulation site is over the tibial or sciatic nerve of the pelvic limb. Because of anatomical restrictions (ie, the carapace), the recording must be made in the cervical region. The author typically has made these recordings in the region of the first cervical vertebra. In this area, a field potential associated with synaptic activity of the ascending spinal tracts (dorsal columns) likely contributes to the waveform seen. To date, this test mainly has been evaluated as an all-or-none phenomenon (ie, waveform present or absent), and although it has shown promise, it needs to be tested more rigorously in a larger group of animals with proper controls before any conclusions can be made.

Electroencephalography

Electroencephalography (EEG) is the recording of electrical activity from the cerebral cortex with electrodes placed on the surface of the head or within the scalp. Numerous electrodes are placed at various points on the head, and the method by which measurements are taken between these electrodes constitutes the EEG montage [202,203]. Unlike many of the electrodiagnostic tests described previously, this is not an evoked response, but a passive recording of intrinsic neuronal activity. The waveforms are produced by synaptic potentials of cerebral cortical neurons, and in mammals, they have typical patterns during different stages of wakefulness and consciousness. These typically are described by their frequency and amplitude. Structural diseases of the brain may produce waveforms of abnormal character (often low-frequency and high-amplitude slow waves). Abnormal, paroxysmal discharges, such as spikes and sharp waves, also can be seen on EEG in animals with epilepsy [202].

In mammalian species, EEG often is recorded with small needle electrodes placed just under the skin. This may be impossible in many reptile patients because of the lack of pliable skin over the head and the presence of scales or scutes. Surface electrodes, however, can be used effectively in these patients with the aid of contact paste (Fig. 10), and recordings can be obtained from reptiles. The small size of some patients may be a limiting factor, as the placement of several electrodes is required to produce the recording.

As with many of the tests described previously, EEG suffers from a lack of clinical studies in normal animals, complicating interpretation, and reports of EEG in reptilian patients are extremely limited [22]. Considerable related work, however, has been done on experimental animals, and this may provide some information that can be extrapolated to clinical patients. EEG of reptiles produces waveforms that are substantially different from mammalian tracings in animals of similar arousal states and consciousness.

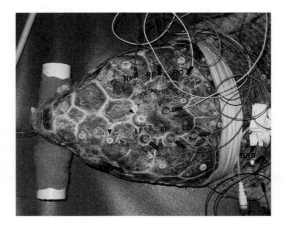

Fig. 10. Electrode placement for electroencephalogram (EEG) recording in a sea turtle that presented in a stuporous state. The recording was made using disk electrodes attached with contact paste at seven points over the skull (identified as left and right frontal [LF and RF, respectively], left and right parietal [LP, RP], left and right occipital [LO, RO] and vertex [V]). A ground electrode (GRD) was placed on the neck. The other disk-shaped structures on the head are barnacles (*arrowheads*). These electrodes ideally would be placed further rostrally for optimal recording.

For example, EEG of reptiles in an aroused state shares many features in common with patterns seen in the slow-wave portion of the mammalian sleep cycle, such as sleep spindles [204,205]. Sharp waves and spikes, suggestive of epileptic activity in mammals, are common findings in EEG recordings from normal reptiles, particularly during quiescent states [205–209]. In fact, reptiles or isolated brain tissue from reptiles (particularly chelonians), are used frequently as experimental models of epileptogenesis [207,210]. These differences must be borne in mind when interpreting recordings from reptilian patients (Fig. 11). As with other electrophysiologic testing, EEG may be altered substantially by the body temperature of the animal at the time of recording [204,209].

Muscle and nerve biopsy

Biopsy and subsequent histopathological evaluation of muscle and nerve tissue are invaluable tools in the identification and diagnosis of diseases affecting the peripheral nerves and muscle tissue. Samples can be collected using techniques identical to those used in more conventional species [211]. Examination of muscle tissue may reveal denervation, inflammatory changes,

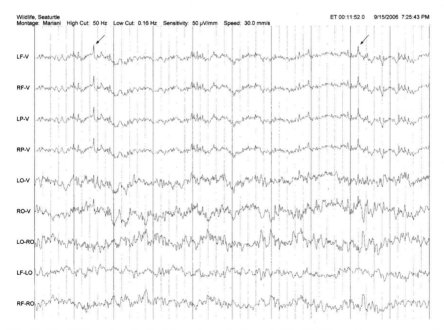

Fig. 11. The EEG tracing obtained from the turtle shown in Fig. 10. This tracing was generated using a combined referential and bipolar montage. Each line represents the electrical difference between two of the electrodes, and is indicated at the left of the figure. Note the large amplitude, paroxysmal spike activity (*arrows*), which may be seen normally in reptiles.

necrosis, or infectious organisms, while nerve histopathology may show evidence of demyelinating disease or axonal degeneration. Submission to a laboratory specializing in this area is recommended, and contacting the laboratory before the collection of samples is usually prudent. Fresh samples often are preferred to formalin-fixed specimens, as they allow for immunohistochemistry and greater characterization of muscle fiber types and pathologic changes.

Acknowledgments

The author acknowledges Drs. Adrienne Atkins, Ramiro Isaza, and Jim Wellehan for case material included in this article. Drs. Jerry Demuth and Kara Sessums helped with performance of some of the electrophysiologic testing shown. The author also thanks Dr. Elliot Jacobson for advice and Dr. Rita Hanel for review of the manuscript.

References

[1] ten Donkelaar HJ. Reptiles. In: Nieuwenhuys R, ten Donkelaar HJ, Nicholson C, editors. The central nervous system of vertebrates, vol. 2. New York: Springer; 1998. p. 1315–524.

[2] Bennett RA, Mehler SJ. Neurology. In: Mader DR, editor. Reptile medicine and surgery. 2nd edition. St. Louis (MO): Saunders Elsevier; 2006. p. 239–50.

[3] Chrisman CL, Walsh M, Meeks JC, et al. Neurologic examination of sea turtles. J Am Vet Med Assoc 1997;211:1043–7.

[4] Keeble E. Neurology. In: Girling SJ, Raiti P, editors. BSAVA manual of reptiles. 2nd edition. Gloucester (MA): British Small Animal Veterinary Association; 2004. p. 273–88.

[5] Schaeffer DO, Waters RM. Neuroanatomy and neurological diseases of reptiles. Seminars in Avian and Exotic Pet Medicine 1996;5:165–71.

[6] Bagley RS. Fundamentals of veterinary clinical neurology. Ames (IA): Blackwell Publishing; 2005. p. 570.

[7] Chrisman CL. Problems in small animal neurology. 2nd edition. Philadelphia: Lea and Febiger; 1991. p. 526.

[8] de Lahunta S. Veterinary neuroanatomy and clinical neurology. 2nd edition. Philadelphia: W.B. Saunders; 1983. p. 471.

[9] Divers SJ. Clinical evaluation of reptiles. Vet Clin North Am Exot Anim Pract 1999;2:291–331.

[10] Frye FL. Biomedical and surgical aspects of captive reptile husbandry. 2nd edition. Malabar (FL): Krieger Publishing Company; 1991. vol. 1. p. 325.

[11] Jacobson ER. Reptiles. Vet Clin North Am Small Anim Pract 1987;17:1203–25.

[12] Lawton MPC. Neurological diseases. In: Benyon PH, Lawton MPC, Cooper JE, editors. BSAVA manual of reptiles. Gloucestershire (UK): British Small Animal Veterinary Association; 1992. p. 128–37.

[13] Rossi JV. General husbandry and management. In: Mader DR, editor. Reptile medicine and surgery. 2nd edition. St. Louis (MO): Saunders Elsevier; 2006. p. 25–41.

[14] Done L. Neurologic disorders. In: Mader DR, editor. Reptile medicine and surgery. 2nd edition. St. Louis (MO): Saunders Elsevier; 2006. p. 852–7.

[15] Norton TM. Chelonian emergency and critical care. Seminars in Avian and Exotic Pet Medicine 2005;14:106–30.

[16] Sadove SS, Pisciotta R, DiGiovanni R. Assessment and initial treatment of cold-stunned sea turtles. Chelonian Conservation and Biology 1998;3:84–6.

[17] Turnbull BS, Smith CR, Stamper MA. Medical implications of hypothermia in threatened Loggerhead (*Caretta caretta*) and endangered Kemp's Ridley (*Lepidochelys kempi*) and green (*Chelonia mydas*) sea turtles. In: Baer CK, Patterson RA, editors. Proceedings of the American Association of Zoo Veterinarians and the International Association for Aquatic Animal Medicine Joint Conference. New Orleans; 2000. p. 31–5.

[18] Bennett RA. Management of common reptile emergencies. In: Frahm MW, editor. Proceedings of the Association of Reptilian and Amphibian Veterinarians. Kansas City (MO); 1998. p. 67–72.

[19] Boyer TH. Common problems and treatment of green iguanas (*Iguana iguana*). Bulletin of the Association of Amphibian and Reptilian Veterinarians 1991;1:8–11.

[20] Boyer TH. Emergency care of reptiles. Seminars in Avian and Exotic Pet Medicine 1994;3: 210–6.

[21] Fowler ME. Metabolic bone disease. In: Fowler ME, editor. Zoo and wild animal medicine. Philadelphia: W.B. Saunders; 1978. p. 55–76.

[22] Frye FL. Biomedical and surgical aspects of captive reptile Husbandry. 2nd edition. Malabar (FL): Krieger Publishing Company; 1991. vol. 2. p. 312.

[23] Jubb TF. A thiamine responsive nervous disease in saltwater crocodiles (*Crocodylus porosus*). Vet Rec 1992;131:347–8.

[24] Boyer TH. Common problems of box turtles (*Terrapene* spp) in captivity. Bulletin of the Association of Reptilian and Amphibian Veterinarians 1992;2:9–14.

[25] O'Malley B. Clinical anatomy and physiology of exotic species: structure and function of mammals, birds, reptiles and amphibians. Philadelphia: Elsevier Saunders; 2005. p. 269.

[26] Willer CJ, Lewbart GA, Lemons C. Aural abscesses in wild eastern box turtles, *Terrapene carolina carolina*, from North Carolina: aerobic bacterial isolates and distribution of lesions. J Herpetol Med Surg 2003;13:4–9.

[27] Farnsworth RJ, Brannian RE, Fletcher KC, et al. A vitamin E-selenium responsive condition in a green iguana. Journal of Zoo Animal Medicine 1986;17:42–3.

[28] Jacobson ER. Evaluation of the reptile patient. In: Jacobson ER, Kollias GV, editors. Contemporary issues in small animal practice: exotic animals. New York: Churchill Livingstone; 1988. p. 1–18.

[29] Borkowski R. Lead poisoning and intestinal perforations in a snapping turtle (*Chelydra serpentina*) due to fishing gear ingestion. J Zoo Wildl Med 1997;28:109–13.

[30] Cooper JE, Jackson OF. Miscellaneous diseases. In: Cooper JE, Jackson OF, editors. Diseases of the reptilia, vol. 2. New York: Academic Press; 1981. p. 487–504.

[31] Lloyd M. Chlorhexidine toxicosis from soaking in red-bellied short-necked turtles, *Emydura subglobosa*. Bulletin of the Association of Reptilian and Amphibian Veterinarians 1996;6(4):6–7.

[32] Holt PE. Drugs and dosages. In: Cooper JE, Jackson OF, editors. Diseases of the reptilia, vol. 2. New York: Academic Press; 1981. p. 551–84.

[33] Jackson OF. Clinical aspects of diagnosis and treatment. In: Cooper JE, Jackson OF, editors. Diseases of the reptilia, vol. 2. New York: Academic Press; 1981. p. 507–34.

[34] Blankenship EL. Suspected intoxication of a loggerhead musk turtle with metronidazole. Bulletin of the Association of Reptilian and Amphibian Veterinarians 1996;6(3):6–7.

[35] Casares M, Enders F. Enrofloxacin side effects in a Galapagos tortoise (*Geochelone elephantopus nigra*). In: Baer CK, editor. Proceedings of the American Association of Zoo Veterinarians. Puerto Vallarta (Mexico); 1996. p. 446–8.

[36] Dumonceaux GA, St. Leger J. Ivermectin intoxication in a group of Nile crocodiles. In: Baer CK, editor. Proceedings of the Association of Reptilian and Amphibian Veterinarians. Naples (FL); 2004. p. 155–7.

[37] Klingenberg RJ. A comparison of fenbendazole and ivermectin for the treatment of nematode parasites in ball pythons, *Python regius*. Bulletin of the Association of Reptilian and Amphibian Veterinarians 1992;2(2):5–6.

[38] Szell Z, Sreter T, Varga I. Ivermectin toxicosis in a chameleon (*Chamaeleo senegalensis*) infected with *Foleyella furcata*. J Zoo Wildl Med 2001;32:115–7.

[39] Teare JA, Bush M. Toxicity and efficacy of ivermectin in chelonians. J Am Vet Med Assoc 1983;183:1195–7.

[40] Barten SL. The medical care of iguanas and other common pet lizards. Vet Clin North Am Small Anim Pract 1993;23:1213–49.

[41] Hernandez-Divers SJ. Clinical aspects of reptile behavior. Vet Clin North Am Exot Anim Pract 2001;4:599–612.

[42] Lock BA. Behavioral and morphologic adaptations. In: Mader DR, editor. Reptile medicine and surgery. 2nd edition. St. Louis (MO): Saunders Elsevier; 2006. p. 163–79.

[43] Jacobson ER. Snakes. Vet Clin North Am Small Anim Pract 1993;23:1179–212.

[44] Wyneken J. Sea turtle locomotion: mechanisms, behavior, and energetics. In: Lutz PL-Musick JA, editors. The biology of sea turtles, vol. 1. New York: CRC Press; 1997. p. 165–98.

[45] Pough FH, Janis CM, Heiser JB. Vertebrate Life. 6th edition. Upper Saddle River (NJ): Prentice Hall; 2002. p. 699.

[46] Isaza R, Garner M, Jacobson E. Proliferative osteoarthritis and osteoarthrosis in 15 snakes. J Zoo Wildl Med 2000;31:20–7.

[47] Schroter M, Heckers KO, Ruschoff B, et al. Severe case of spinal osteomyelitis due to Enterococcus spp. in a three-year old rhinoceros horned viper, Bitis nasicornis. J Herpetol Med Surg 2005;15(3):53–6.

[48] Hernandez-Divers SJ. Diagnostic techniques. In: Mader DR, editor. Reptile medicine and surgery. 2nd edition. St. Louis (MO): Saunders Elsevier; 2006. p. 490–532.

[49] Molenaar GJ. Anatomy and physiology of infrared sensitivity of snakes. In: Gans C, editor. Biology of the reptilia, vol. 17. Chicago: University of Chicago Press; 1992. p. 367–453.

[50] Burghardt GM. Chemical perception in reptiles. In: Johnston JW, Moulton DG, Turk A, editors. Advances in chemoreception I. Communication by chemical signals, vol. 1. New York: Appleton Century Crofts; 1970. p. 241–308.

[51] Eisthen HL. Evolution of vertebrate olfactory systems. Brain Behav Evol 1997;50:222–33.

[52] Jacobson ER, Klingenberg RJ, Homer BL, et al. Inclusion body disease (Roundtable). Bulletin of the Association of Reptilian and Amphibian Veterinarians 1999;9(2):18–25.

[53] McNamara TS, Cook RA, Behler JL, et al. Cryptococcosis in a common anaconda (Eunectes murinus). J Zoo Wildl Med 1994;25:128–32.

[54] Lawton MPC. Reptilian ophthalmology. In: Mader DR, editor. Reptile medicine and surgery. 2nd edition. St. Louis (MO): Saunders Elsevier; 2006. p. 323–42.

[55] Nevarez JG, Mitchell MA, Kim DY, et al. West Nile virus in alligator, Alligator mississippiensis, ranches from Louisiana. J Herpetol Med Surg 2005;15(3):4–9.

[56] Kardong KV. Vertebrates: comparative anatomy, function, evolution. 4th edition. New York: McGraw Hill; 2006. p. 782.

[57] Evans HE. Introduction and anatomy. In: Fowler ME, editor. Zoo and wild animal medicine. Philadelphia: W.B. Saunders; 1978. p. 91–113.

[58] Crowe A. Muscle spindles, tendon organs, and joint receptors. In: Gans C, editor. Biology of the reptilia, vol. 17. Chicago: University of Chicago Press; 1992. p. 454–95.

[59] Mortin LI, Stein PS. Spinal cord segments containing key elements of the central pattern generators for three forms of scratch reflex in the turtle. J Neurosci 1989;9:2285–96.

[60] Robertson GA, Mortin LI, Keifer J, et al. Three forms of the scratch reflex in the spinal turtle: central generation of motor patterns. J Neurophysiol 1985;53:1517–34.

[61] Cruce WLR. Spinal cord in lizards. In: Gans C, Northcutt RG, Ulinski P, editors. Biology of the Reptilia: neurology B, vol. 10. New York: Academic Press; 1979. p. 111–31.

[62] Srivastava VK. Functional recovery following reptilean (Calotus calotus) spinal cord transection. Indian J Physiol Pharmacol 1992;36:193–6.

[63] Davies PMC. Anatomy and physiology. In: Cooper JE, Jackson OF, editors. Diseases of the reptilia, vol. 1. New York: Academic Press; 1981. p. 9–73.

[64] Heard D, Harr K, Wellehan J. Diagnostic sampling and laboratory tests. In: Girling SJ, Raiti P, editors. BSAVA manual of reptiles. 2nd edition. Gloucester (UK): British Small Animal Veterinary Association; 2004. p. 71–86.

[65] Gyimesi ZS, Garner MM, Burns RB, et al. High incidence of lymphoid neoplasia in a colony of Egyptian spiny-tailed lizards (*Uromastyx aegyptius*). J Zoo Wildl Med 2005;36: 103–10.

[66] Schultze AE, Mason GL, Clyde VL. Lymphosarcoma with leukemic blood profile in a Savannah monitor lizard (*Varanus exanthematicus*). J Zoo Wildl Med 1999;30: 158–64.

[67] Mader DR. Nutritional secondary hyperparathyroidism in green iguanas. In: Bonagura JD, editor. Kirk's current veterinary therapy XIII small animal practice. Philadelphia: W.B. Saunders; 2000. p. 1179–82.

[68] Wallach JD. Feeding and nutritional diseases. In: Fowler ME, editor. Zoo and wild animal medicine. Philadelphia: W.B. Saunders; 1978. p. 123–8.

[69] Raiti P. Uraemic encephalopathy in a leaf-tailed gecko (*Uroplatus henkeli*). In: Baer CK, editor. Proceedings of the Association of Reptilian and Amphibian Veterinarians. Reno (NV); 2000. p. 29–30.

[70] Garner MM, Lung NP, Murray S. Xanthomatosis in geckos: five cases. J Zoo Wildl Med 1999;30:443–7.

[71] Gyimesi ZS, Stedman NL, Crossett VR. Cholesterol granulomas in a great plated lizard, *Gerrhosaurus major*. J Herpetol Med Surg 2002;12(3):36–9.

[72] McBride M, Koch TF, Hernandez-Divers S, et al. Preliminary evaluation of resting and postprandial bile acid levels and a novel biliverdin assay in the green iguana (Iguana iguana). In: Baer CK, editor. Proceedings of the Association of Reptilian and Amphibian Veterinarians. Naples (FL); 2004. p. 105 [abstract].

[73] Redrobe S, MacDonald J. Sample collection and clinical pathology of reptiles. Vet Clin North Am Exot Anim Pract 1999;2:709–30.

[74] Chitty JR. Lead toxicosis in a Greek tortoise (*Testudo graeca*). In: Baer CK, editor. Proceedings of the Association of Reptilian and Amphibian Veterinarians. Minneapolis (MN); 2003. p. 101 [abstract].

[75] Girling SJ, Fraser MA. *Listeria monocytogenes* septicaemia in an inland bearded dragon, *Pogona vitticeps*. J Herpetol Med Surg 2004;14(3):6–9.

[76] Ramsay EC, Daniel GB, Tryon BW, et al. Osteomyelitis associated with *Salmonella enterica* SS arizonae in a colony of ridgenose rattlesnakes (*Crotalus willardi*). J Zoo Wildl Med 2002;33:301–10.

[77] Berry KH, Brown DR, Brown M, et al. Reptilian mycoplasmal infections (roundtable). J Herpetol Med Surg 2002;12(3):8–20.

[78] Clippinger TL, Bennett RA, Johnson CM, et al. *Mycoplasma epizootic* in a herd of bull alligators (*Alligator mississippiensis*). In: Baer CK, editor. Proceedings of the American Association of Zoo Veterinarians. Puerto Vallarta (Mexico); 1996. p. 230–4.

[79] Frye FL, Munn RJ, Gardner M, et al. Adenovirus-like hepatitis in a group of related Rankin's dragon lizards (*Pogona henrylawsoni*). J Zoo Wildl Med 1994;25:167–71.

[80] Jacobson ER. Viral diseases of reptiles. In: Fowler ME, Miller RE, editors. Zoo & wild animal medicine: Current therapy 4. Philadelphia: W.B. Saunders; 1999. p. 153–9.

[81] Jacobson ER. West Nile virus infection in crocodilians. In: Baer CK, editor. Proceedings of the Association of Reptilian and Amphibian Veterinarians. Naples (FL); 2004. p. 85–6.

[82] Jacobson ER, Flanagan JP, Rideout B, et al. Ophidian paramyxovirus (roundtable). Bulletin of the Association of Reptilian and Amphibian Veterinarians 1999;9(1):15–22.

[83] Jacobson ER, Gaskin JM, Gardiner CH. Adenovirus-like infection in a boa constrictor. J Am Vet Med Assoc 1985;187:1226–7.

[84] Jacobson ER, Gaskin JM, Wells S, et al. Epizootic of ophidian paramyxovirus in a zoological collection: pathological, microbiological, and serological findings. J Zoo Wildl Med 1992;23:318–27.

[85] Jacobson ER, Troutman JM, Ginn P, et al. Outbreak of West Nile virus in farmed alligators (*Alligator mississippiensis*) in Florida. In: Baer CK, editor. Proceedings of the Association of Reptilian and Amphibian Veterinarians. Minneapolis (MN); 2003. p. 3 [abstract].

[86] Kim DY, Mitchell MA, Bauer RW, et al. An outbreak of adenoviral infection in inland bearded dragons (*Pogona vitticeps*) coinfected with dependovirus and coccidial protozoa (Isospora sp.). J Vet Diagn Invest 2002;14:332–4.

[87] McArthur S, Blahak S, Koelle P, et al. Chelonian herpesvirus (roundtable). J Herpetol Med Surg 2002;12(2):14–31.

[88] Schumacher J. Selected infectious diseases of wild reptiles and amphibians. Journal of Exotic Pet Medicine 2006;15:18–24.

[89] Schumacher J. Viral diseases of reptiles. In: Bonagura JD, editor. Kirk's current veterinary therapy XIII small animal practice. Philadelphia: W.B. Saunders; 2000. p. 1174–6.

[90] Wellehan JF, Johnson AJ. Reptile virology. Vet Clin North Am Exot Anim Pract 2005;8: 27–52.

[91] West G, Garner M, Raymond J, et al. Meningoencephalitis in a Boelen's python (*Morelia boeleni*) associated with paramyxovirus infection. J Zoo Wildl Med 2001;32:360–5.

[92] Fleming GJ, Heard DJ, Jacobson E, et al. Cytoplasmic inclusions in corn snakes, *Elaphe guttata*, resembling inclusion body disease of boid snakes. J Herpetol Med Surg 2003; 13(2):18–22.

[93] Jacobson ER, Oros J, Tucker SJ, et al. Partial characterization of retroviruses from boid snakes with inclusion body disease. Am J Vet Res 2001;62:217–24.

[94] Schumacher J, Jacobson ER, Homer BL, et al. Inclusion body disease in boid snakes. J Zoo Wildl Med 1994;25:511–24.

[95] Holz PH, Slocombe R. Systemic fusarium infection in two snakes, carpet python, *Morelia spilota variegata* and a red-bellied black snake, *Pseudechis porphyriacus*. J Herpetol Med Surg 2000;10(2):18–20.

[96] Manharth A, Lemberger K, Mylniczenko N, et al. Disseminated phaeohyphomycosis due to an *Exophiala* species in a Galopagos tortoise, *Geochelone nigra*. J Herpetol Med Surg 2005;15(2):20–6.

[97] Migaki G, Jacobson ER, Casey HW. Fungal diseases in reptiles. In: Hoff GL, Frye FL, Jacobson ER, editors. Diseases of amphibians and reptiles. New York: Plenum Press; 1984. p. 183–204.

[98] Williams LW, Jacobson E, Gelatt KN, et al. Phycomycosis in a western massasauga rattlesnake (*Sistrurus catenatus*) with infection of the telencephalon, orbit, and facial structures. Vet Med Small Anim Clin 1979;74:1181–4.

[99] Barnard SM, Upton SJ. A veterinary guide to the parasites of reptiles: protozoa. Malabar (FL): Krieger Publishing Company; 1994. vol. 1. p. 154.

[100] Frank W. Non-hemoparasitic protozoans. In: Hoff GL, Frye FL, Jacobson ER, editors. Diseases of reptiles and amphibians. New York: Plenum Press; 1984. p. 259–384.

[101] Hollamby S, Creeper J. Sarcocystis-like parasite in a black headed monitor, *Varanus tristis tristis*. Bulletin of the Association of Reptilian and Amphibian Veterinarians 1997;7(2): 6–7.

[102] Jacobson ER, Homer BL, Stacy BA, et al. Neurological disease in wild loggerhead sea turtles *Caretta caretta*. Dis Aquat Org 2006;70:139–54.

[103] Johnson CA, Griffith JW, Tenorio P, et al. Fatal trematodiasis in research turtles. Lab Anim Sci 1998;48:340–3.

[104] Jacobson E. Laboratory investigations. In: Benyon PH, Lawton MPC, Cooper JE, editors. BSAVA manual of reptiles. Gloucestershire (UK): British Small Animal Veterinary Association; 1992. p. 50–62.

[105] Westfall ME, Demcovitz DL, Plourde DR, et al. In vitro antibiotic susceptibility of *Mycoplasma iguanae* proposed sp. nov. isolated from vertebral lesions of green iguanas (*Iguana iguana*). J Zoo Wildl Med 2006;37:206–8.

[106] Jacobson ER, Johnson AJ, Hernandez JA, et al. Validation and use of an indirect enzyme-linked immunosorbent assay for detection of antibodies to West Nile virus in American Alligators (*Alligator mississippiensis*) in Florida. J Wildl Dis 2005;41:107–14.

[107] Jacobson ER, Bissell ZK, Arai M. An update on inclusion body disease of boid snakes. In: Baer CK, editor. Proceedings of the Association of Reptilian and Amphibian Veterinarians. Naples (FL); 2004. p. 126–7.

[108] Lock BA, Jacobson E. Use of an ELISA to survey exposure of wild caught boa constrictors, *Boa constrictor*, to retroviruses isolated from boids with inclusion body disease. J Herpetol Med Surg 2005;15(2):4–8.

[109] Garner MM, Raymond JT. Methods for diagnosing inclusion body disease in snakes. In: Baer CK, editor. Proceedings of the Association of Reptilian and Amphibian Veterinarians. Naples (FL); 2004. p. 21–5.

[110] Lennox AM. Equipment for exotic mammal and reptile diagnostics and surgery. Journal of Exotic Pet Medicine 2006;15:98–105.

[111] Marschang RE, Chitty J. Infectious diseases. In: Girling SJ, Raiti P, editors. BSAVA manual of reptiles. 2nd edition. Gloucester (MA): British Small Animal Veterinary Association; 2004. p. 330–45.

[112] Origgi FC, Klein PA, Tucker SJ, et al. Application of immunoperoxidase-based techniques to detect herpesvirus infection in tortoises. J Vet Diagn Invest 2003;15:133–40.

[113] Bennett RA. Neurology. In: Mader DR, editor. Reptile medicine and surgery. Philadelphia: W.B. Saunders Company; 1996. p. 141–8.

[114] Clippinger TL, Bennett RA, Johnson CM, et al. Morbidity and mortality associated with a new mycoplasma species from captive American alligators (*Alligator mississippiensis*). J Zoo Wildl Med 2000;31:303–14.

[115] Owens DW, Ruiz G. New methods of obtaining blood and cerebrospinal fluid from marine turtles. Herpetologica 1980;36:17–20.

[116] Schilliger L. Les affections du systeme nerveux central chez les ophidiens 2-Etude clinique. Le Point Veterinaire 1999;30:41–8.

[117] Whitaker BR, Krum H. Medical management of sea turtles in aquaria. In: Fowler ME, Miller RE, editors. Zoo & wild animal medicine: current therapy 4. Philadelphia: W.B. Saunders; 1999. p. 217–31.

[118] Jacobson ER. Blood collection techniques in reptiles: laboratory investigations. In: Fowler ME, Miller RE, editors. Zoo & wild animal medicine: current therapy 4. Philadelphia: W.B. Saunders; 1999. p. 144–52.

[119] Frye FL. Reptile clinician's handbook: a compact clinical and surgical reference. Malabar (FL): Krieger Publishing Company; 1995. p. 276.

[120] Bennett RA, Hart SH, McSherry LJ, et al. Analysis of cerebrospinal fluid in the American Alligator. In: BSAVA Congress: scientific proceedings. Gloucester, UK: British Small Animal Veterinary Association (BSAVA); 2001. p. 554

[121] Brown DR, Farley JM, Zacher LA, et al. *Mycoplasma alligatoris* sp. nov., from American alligators. Int J Syst Evol Microbiol 2001;51:419–24.

[122] Hernandez-Divers SM, Orcutt CJ, Stahl SJ, et al. Lymphoma in lizards: three case reports. J Herpetol Med Surg 2003;13(1):14–22.

[123] Suedmeyer WK, Turk JR. Lymphoblastic leukemia in an inland bearded dragon, *Pogona vitticeps*. Bulletin of the Association of Reptilian and Amphibian Veterinarians 1996;6(4): 10–2.

[124] DeShaw B, Schoenfeld A, Cook RA, et al. Imaging of reptiles: a comparison study of various radiographic techniques. J Zoo Wildl Med 1996;27:364–70.

[125] Jackson OF, Sainsbury AW. Radiological and related investigations. In: Benyon PH, Lawton MPC, Cooper JE, editors. BSAVA manual of reptiles. Gloucestershire (UK): British Small Animal Veterinary Association; 1992. p. 63–72.

[126] Mitchell MA. Diagnosis and management of reptile orthopedic injuries. Vet Clin North Am Exot Anim Pract 2002;5:97–114.

[127] Raiti P. Non-invasive imaging. In: Girling SJ, Raiti P, editors. BSAVA manual of reptiles. 2nd edition. Gloucester (MA): British small animal veterinary association; 2004. p. 87–102.

[128] Rubel GA, Isenbugel E, Wolvekamp P, editors. An atlas of diagnostic radiology of exotic pets. Philadelphia: W.B. Saunders; 1991. p. 224.

[129] Schumacher J, Toal RL. Advanced radiography and ultrasonography in reptiles. Seminars in Avian and Exotic Pet Medicine 2001;10:162–8.

[130] Silverman S. Diagnostic imaging. In: Mader DR, editor. Reptile medicine and surgery. 2nd edition. St. Louis (MO): Saunders Elsevier; 2006. p. 471–81.

[131] Silverman S. Diagnostic imaging of exotic pets. Vet Clin North Am Small Anim Pract 1993; 23:1287–99.

[132] Stetter MD. Diagnostic imaging of reptiles. In: Bonagura JD, editor. Kirk's current veterinary therapy XIII small animal practice. Philadelphia: W.B. Saunders; 2000. p. 1163–8.

[133] Stoskopf MK. Clinical imaging in zoological medicine: a review. J Zoo Wildl Med 1989;20: 396–412.

[134] Frye FL. Traumatic and physical diseases. In: Cooper JE, Jackson OF, editors. Diseases of the reptilia, vol. 2. New York: Academic Press; 1981. p. 387–407.

[135] Kelly T, Sleeman J. Eastern painted turtle, *Chrysemys picta* (What's your diagnosis?). Journal of Herpetological Medicine and Surgery 2002;12(1):33–5.

[136] Parr KA, Gamble KC, Kinsel M. What's your diagnosis? J Herpetol Med Surg 2005;15(4): 28–30.

[137] Divers SJ, Lawton MPC. Spinal osteomyelitis in a green iguana, *Iguana iguana*: cerebrospinal fluid and myelogram diagnosis. In: Baer CK, editor. Proceedings of the Association of Reptilian and Amphibian Veterinarians. Reno (NV); 2000. p. 77.

[138] Hudson JA, Finn-Bodner ST, Steiss JE. Neurosonography. Vet Clin North Am Small Anim Pract 1998;28:943–72.

[139] Hernandez-Divers SJ, Strunk A, Frank PM, et al. Scintigraphic imaging of a Horsfields tortoise, *Testudo horsfieldi*, with multifocal bacterial and fungal infections, and plastron necrosis. In: Bradley T, editor. Proceedings of the Association of Reptilian and Amphibian Veterinarians. Reno (NV); 2002. p. 103–4

[140] Smith CR, Turnbull BS, Osborn AL, et al. Bone scintigraphy and computed tomography: advanced diagnostic imaging techniques in endangered sea turtles. In: Baer CK, Patterson RA, editors. Proceedings of the American Association of Zoo Veterinarinas and International Association for Aquatic Animal Medicine Joint Conference. New Orleans (LA); 2000. p. 217–21.

[141] Abou-Madi N, Hernandez-Divers SM, Scrivani PV, et al. Computed tomography of pectoral girdle injuries in two chelonians. In: Baer CK, Willette MM, editors. Proceedings of the American Association of Zoo Veterinarians, American Association of Wildlife Veterinarians, Association of Reptilian and Amphibian Veterinarians and National Association of Zoo and Wildlife Veterinarians joint conference. Orlando (FL); 2001. p. 6–9.

[142] Abou-Madi N, Scrivani PV, Kollias GV, et al. Diagnosis of skeletal injuries in chelonians using computed tomography. J Zoo Wildl Med 2004;35:226–31.

[143] Gumpenberger M. Computed tomography (CT) in chelonians. In: Bradley T, editor. Proceedings of the Association of Reptilian and Amphibian Veterinarians. Reno (NV); 2002. p. 41–4.

[144] Gumpenberger M, Henninger W. The use of computed tomography in avian and reptile medicine. Seminars in Avian and Exotic Pet Medicine 2001;10:174–80.

[145] Mathes KA, Fehr M. The use of computed tomography as a diagnostic tool in reptile practice: Selected cases. In: Baer CK, editor. Proceedings of the Association of Reptilian and Amphibian Veterinarians. Minneapolis (MN); 2003. p. 24–7.

[146] Raiti P. The use of computerized tomography and magnetic resonance imaging in chelonian medicine. In: Frahm MW, editor. Proceedings of the Association of Reptilian and Amphibian Veterinarians. Kansas City (MO); 1998. p. 51–4.

[147] Raiti P, Haramati N. Magnetic resonance imaging and computerized tomography of a gravid leopard tortoise (*Geochelone pardalis pardalis*) with metabolic bone disease. J Zoo Wildl Med 1997;28:189–97.

[148] Rubel A, Kuoni W, Augustiny N. Emerging techniques: CT scan and MRI in reptile medicine. Seminars in Avian and Exotic Pet Medicine 1994;3:156–60.

[149] Spaulding K, Loomis MR. Principles and applications of computed tomography and magnetic resonance imaging in zoo and wildlife medicine. In: Fowler ME, Miller RE, editors. Zoo & wild animal medicine: current therapy 4. Philadelphia: W.B. Saunders; 1999. p. 83–8.

[150] Stetter MD, Raphael BL, Haramati N, et al. Comparison of magnetic resonance imaging, computerized axial tomography, ultrasonography and radiology for reptilian diagnostic imaging. In: Baer CK, editor. Proceedings of the American Association of Zoo Veterinarians. Puerto Vallarta (Mexico); 1996. p. 450–53.

[151] Valente AL, Cuenca R, Parga ML, et al. Cervical and coelomic radiologic features of the loggerhead sea turtle, Caretta caretta. Can J Vet Res 2006;70:285–90.

[152] Straub J, Jurina K. Magnetic resonance imaging in chelonians. Seminars in Avian and Exotic Pet Medicine 2001;10:181–6.

[153] Anderson CL, Kabalka GW, Layne DG, et al. Noninvasive high field MRI brain imaging of the garter snake (Thamnophis sirtalis). Copeia 2000;265–9.

[154] Croft LA, Graham JP, Schaf SA, et al. Evaluation of magnetic resonance imaging for detection of internal tumors in green turtles with cutaneous fibropapillomatosis. J Am Vet Med Assoc 2004;225:1428–35.

[155] Valente AL, Cuenca R, Zamora MA, et al. Sectional anatomic and magnetic resonance imaging features of coelomic structures of loggerhead sea turtles. Am J Vet Res 2006;67: 1347–53.

[156] Schmidt RE, Hubbard GB. Atlas of zoo animal pathology. Boca Raton (FL): CRC Press; 1987. vol. 2. p. 117.

[157] Craig LE, Wolf JC, Ramsay EC. Spinal cord glioma in a ridge-nosed rattlesnake (Crotalus willardi). J Zoo Wildl Med 2005;36:313–5.

[158] Garner MM, Hernandez-Divers SM, Raymond JT. Reptile neoplasia: a retrospective study of case submissions to a specialty diagnostic service. Vet Clin North Am Exot Anim Pract 2004;7:653–71.

[159] Cooper JE, Jackson OF, Harshbarger JC. A neurilemmal sarcoma in a tortoise (Testudo hermanni). J Comp Pathol 1983;93:541–5.

[160] Diaz-Figueroa O, Toomey J, Mitchell MA, et al. Peripheral nerve sheath tumor in the coelomic cavity of a Savannah monitor (Varanus exanthematicus). In: Baer CK, editor. Proceedings of the Association of Reptilian and Amphibian Veterinarians. Naples (FL); 2004. p. 135–7.

[161] Effron M, Griner L, Benirschke K. Nature and rate of neoplasia found in captive wild mammals, birds, and reptiles at necropsy. J Natl Cancer Inst 1977;59:185–98.

[162] Linn MJ, Steinberg JJ, Kress Y. Pituitary adenoma in a black-headed python (Aspidites melanocephalus). In: Baer CK, editor. Proceedings of the American Association of Zoo Veterinarians. Puerta Vallarta (Mexico); 1996. p. 449 [abstract].

[163] Mikaelian I, Levine BS, Smith SG, et al. Malignant peripheral nerve sheath tumor in a bearded dragon, Pogona vitticeps. J Herpetol Med Surg 2001;11(1):9–12.

[164] Ramis A, Pumarola M, Fernandez-Moran J, et al. Malignant peripheral nerve sheath tumor in a water moccasin (Agkistrodon piscivorus). J Vet Diagn Invest 1998;10:205–8.

[165] Schmidt RE, Hubbard GB, Fletcher KC. Systematic survey of lesions from animals in a zoologic collection: I. Central nervous system. Journal of Zoo Animal Medicine 1986; 17:8–11.

[166] Scott HH, Beattie J. Neoplasm in a porose crocodile with an addendum. J Pathol Bacteriol 1927;30:61–6.

[167] Catao-Dias JL, Nichols DK. Neoplasia in snakes at the national zoological park, Washington, DC (1978–1997). J Comp Pathol 1999;120:89–95.

[168] Griner LA. Pathology of zoo animals. San Diego (CA): Zoological Society of San Diego; 1983. p. 608.

[169] Harshbarger JC. Neoplasms in zoo poikilotherms emphasizing cases in the registry of tumors in lower animals. In: Montali RJ, Migaki G, editors. Comparative pathology of zoo animals. Washington, DC: Smithsonian Institution Press; 1978. p. 585–91.

[170] Jacobson ER. Neoplastic diseases. In: Cooper JE, Jackson OF, editors. Diseases of the reptilia, vol. 2. New York: Academic Press; 1981. p. 429–68.

[171] Machotka SV. Neoplasia in reptiles. In: Hoff GL, Frye FL, Jacobson E, editors. Diseases of amphibians and reptiles. New York: Plenum Press; 1984. p. 519–80.

[172] Machotka SV, Whitney GD. Neoplasms in snakes: report of a probable mesothelioma in a rattlesnake and a thorough tabulation of earlier cases. In: Montali RJ, Migaki G, editors. Comparative pathology of zoo animals. Washington, DC: Smithsonian Institution Press; 1978. p. 593–602.

[173] Montali RJ. An overview of tumors in zoo animals. In: Montali RJ, Migaki G, editors. Comparative pathology of zoo animals. Washington, DC: Smithsonian Institution Press; 1978. p. 531–42.

[174] Ramsay EC, Munson L, Lowenstine L, et al. A retrospective study of neoplasia in a collection of captive snakes. J Zoo Wildl Med 1996;27:28–34.

[175] Dawe CJ, Banfield WG, Small JD, et al. Chondrosarcoma of a corn snake and nephroblastoma of a rainbow trout in cell culture. In: Montali RJ, Migaki G, editors. Comparative pathology of zoo animals. Washington, DC: Smithsonian Institution Press; 1978. p. 603–12.

[176] McNulty E, Hoffman R. Fibrosarcoma in a corn snake, *Elaphe guttata*. Bulletin of the Association of Reptilian and Amphibian Veterinarians 1995;5:7–8.

[177] Wadsworth JR. Some neoplasms of captive wild animals. J Am Vet Med Assoc 1954;125: 121–3.

[178] Sims MH. Clinical electrodiagnostic evaluation in exotic animal medicine. Seminars in Avian and Exotic Pet Medicine 1996;5:140–9.

[179] Chrisman CL, Burt JK, Wood PK, et al. Electromyography in small animal clinical neurology. J Am Vet Med Assoc 1972;160:311–8.

[180] Niederhauser UB, Holliday TA. Electrodiagnostic studies in diseases of muscles and neuromuscular junctions. Semin Vet Med Surg (Small Anim) 1989;4:116–25.

[181] Sims MH. Electrodiagnostic techniques in the evaluation of diseases affecting skeletal muscle. Vet Clin North Am Small Anim Pract 1983;13:145–62.

[182] Walker TL, Redding RW, Braund KG. Motor nerve conduction velocity and latency in the dog. Am J Vet Res 1979;40:1433–9.

[183] Lee AF, Bowen JM. Effect of tissue temperature on ulnar nerve conduction velocity in the dog. Am J Vet Res 1975;36:1305–7.

[184] Steiss JE, Marshall AE. Electromyographic evaluation of conduction time and velocity of the recurrent laryngeal nerves of clinically normal dogs. Am J Vet Res 1988;49: 1533–6.

[185] Whalen LR, Spurgeon TL. Trigeminal nerve-evoked potentials in the dog. Am J Vet Res 1986;47:2435–40.

[186] Cuddon PA. Electrodiagnosis in veterinary neurology: electromyography, nerve conduction studies, and evoked potentials. 2006.

[187] Knecht CD, Redding R, Hyams D. Stimulation techniques and response characteristics of the M and F waves and H reflex in dogs. Vet Res Commun 1983;6:123–32.

[188] Sims MH, McLean RA. Use of repetitive nerve stimulation to assess neuromuscular function in dogs. A test protocol or suspected myasthenia gravis. Progress in Veterinary Neurology 1990;1:311–9.

[189] Sims MH, Moore RE. Auditory-evoked response in the clinically normal dog: early latency components. Am J Vet Res 1984;45:2019–27.

[190] Marshall AE. Brain stem auditory-evoked response of the nonanesthetized dog. Am J Vet Res 1985;46:966–73.

[191] Sims MH. Electrodiagnostic evaluation of auditory function. Vet Clin North Am Small Anim Pract 1988;18:913–44.

[192] Munro KJ, Paul B, Cox CL. Normative auditory brainstem response data for bone conduction in the dog. J Small Anim Pract 1997;38:353–6.

[193] Strain GM, Tedford BL, Littlefield-Chabaud MA, et al. Air- and bone-conduction brainstem auditory evoked potentials and flash visual evoked potentials in cats. Am J Vet Res 1998;59:135–7.

[194] Baird IL. The anatomy of the reptilian ear. In: Gans C, editor. Biology of the reptilia, vol. 2. New York: Academic Press; 1978. p. 193–275.

[195] Hartline PH. Physiological basis for detection of sound and vibration in snakes. J Exp Biol 1971;54:349–71.

[196] Hartline PH. Midbrain responses of the auditory and somatic vibration systems in snakes. J Exp Biol 1971;54:373–90.

[197] Corwin JT, Bullock TH, Schweitzer J. The auditory brain stem response in five vertebrate classes. Electroencephalogr Clin Neurophysiol 1982;54:629–41.

[198] Bartol SM, Musick JA, Lenhardt ML. Auditory evoked potentials of the loggerhead sea turtle (*Caretta caretta*). Copeia 1999;836–40.

[199] Holliday TA. Electrodiagnostic examination. Somatosensory evoked potentials and electromyography. Vet Clin North Am Small Anim Pract 1992;22:833–57.

[200] Holliday TA, Weldon NE, Ealand BG. Percutaneous recording of evoked spinal cord potentials of dogs. Am J Vet Res 1979;40:326–33.

[201] Poncelet L, Michaux C, Balligand M. Study of spinal cord evoked injury potential by use of computer modeling and in dogs with naturally acquired thoracolumbar spinal cord compression. Am J Vet Res 1998;59:300–6.

[202] Holliday TA, Williams DC. Interictal paroxysmal discharges in the electroencephalograms of epileptic dogs. Clin Tech Small Anim Pract 1998;13:132–43.

[203] Redding RW, Knecht CE. Atlas of electroencephalography in the dog and cat. New York: Praeger; 1984. p. 400.

[204] De Vera L, Gonzalez J, Rial RV. Reptilian waking EEG: slow waves, spindles, and evoked potentials. Electroencephalogr Clin Neurophysiol 1994;90:298–303.

[205] Flanigan WF Jr. Sleep and wakefulness in iguanid lizards, *Ctenosaura pectinata* and *Iguana iguana*. Brain Behav Evol 1973;8:401–36.

[206] Gaztelu JM, Garcia-Austt E, Bullock TH. Electrocorticograms of hippocampal and dorsal cortex of two reptiles: comparison with possible mammalian homologs. Brain Behav Evol 1991;37:144–60.

[207] Russo RE, Velluti JC. Inhibitory effects of excitatory amino acids on pyramidal cells of the in vitro turtle medial cortex. Exp Brain Res 1992;92:85–93.

[208] Velluti JC, Russo RE, Simini F, et al. Electroencephalogram in vitro and cortical transmembrane potentials in the turtle *Chrysemys d'orbigny*. Brain Behav Evol 1991;38:7–19.

[209] Walker JM, Berger RJ. A polygraphic study of the tortoise (*Testudo denticulata*). Absence of electrophysiological signs of sleep. Brain Behav Evol 1973;8:453–67.

[210] Servit Z, Strejckova A. Influence of nasal respiration upon normal EEG and epileptic electrographic activities in frog and turtle. Physiol Bohemoslov 1976;25:109–14.

[211] Dickinson PJ, LeCouteur RA. Muscle and nerve biopsy. Vet Clin North Am Small Anim Pract 2002;32:63–102.

VETERINARY
CLINICS
Exotic Animal Practice

Vet Clin Exot Anim 10 (2007) 893–907

Principles of Neurological Imaging of Exotic Animal Species

Marguerite F. Knipe, DVM, DACVIM (Neurology)

Department of Surgical and Radiological Sciences, School of Veterinary Medicine,
University of California–Davis, 2122 Tupper Hall, Davis, CA 95616, USA

The most obvious difficulty with imaging the central nervous system (CNS) in any species is that it is encased almost entirely in bone, limiting the means by which the clinician can evaluate it. Additionally, in many companion exotic species, their small size further complicates diagnostic evaluation of the brain and spinal cord. Knowledge of the advantages and limitations of different imaging modalities, along with the neuroanatomical localization and assessment of likely causes of disease, will permit the clinician to choose the most appropriate imaging method for the patient. There are several excellent references describing species-specific restraint and positioning, as well as imaging atlases, and the reader is directed to these in other portions of this article. This article discusses the basic imaging principles of radiology, myelography, CT, and MRI of the nervous system of companion exotic animals, to aid exotic animal clinicians in selecting imaging modalities and interpreting the results.

Localizing the lesion for imaging purposes

Before proceeding with any type of imaging, the clinician must be sure he or she is evaluating the appropriate area of the CNS. A thorough neurological examination is necessary to permit localization of a lesion to one (or more) of the main divisions of the nervous system: brain, spinal cord, or neuromuscular system. A patient presenting with tetraparesis could have brain disease, cervical spinal cord disease, or even generalized neuromuscular disease. The diagnostic plan for each of these localizations is very different, and it is the duty of the clinician to ensure that the patient is not placed at risk, and the client's money is not spent on potentially unnecessary procedures. Although basic neuroanatomy is similar across species,

E-mail address: mfknipe@ucdavis.edu

doi:10.1016/j.cvex.2007.05.001

knowledge of the specific differences between exotic animals is crucial for exotic animal clinicians, as the variety of species they evaluate is often much wider than that of small and large animal veterinarians.

Radiography

Radiographic evaluation of the skull and vertebral column is the most economic and readily available imaging modality to the exotic animal clinician, and several publications describe restraint, positioning, and normal radiographic anatomy [1–4]. Unfortunately, radiographic evaluation of the CNS only will provide information about skeletal abnormalities, and cannot definitely provide the clinician with information about the neural structures. If the patient presents for paraplegia, and radiographic images show a vertebral fracture, one can assume that the neurological deficits are secondary to the vertebral lesion, but this cannot be proven without additional diagnostic testing. Abnormalities that are most likely to be seen on radiographs are:

  Osteoproduction—hyperostosis, spondylosis, discospondylitis, osteomyelitis [5], osteoarthrosis [6], neoplasia
  Osteolysis—metabolic bone disease (plus or minus pathologic fracture), discospondylitis, osteomyelitis, neoplasia [7]
  Fracture/luxation—secondary to trauma, metabolic bone disease, or neoplasia
  Congenital bony anomalies—scoliosis, kyphosis, vertebral anomalies (eg, hemivertebrae, butterfly vertebrae, spina bifida)
  Metallic foreign bodies

Proper patient positioning and exposure technique are important for reliable interpretation of the radiographic images. Recent advances in digital radiography permit some leeway in radiographic exposure technique, but poorly exposed or poorly positioned radiographs can either mask or mimic potential lesions.

A complete radiographic survey study of the skull includes lateral, ventrodorsal (VD) (Fig. 1), and two oblique projections (plus or minus open-mouthed view). A complete radiographic evaluation of the vertebral column includes at least two orthogonal views (lateral and VD), and occasionally oblique or dynamic views (flexion or extension). If trauma to the vertebral column is known or suspected, lateral radiographic views should be evaluated first, before ventrodorsal views are obtained, to minimize manipulation and avoid possible exacerbation of a traumatic lesion. General anesthesia or heavy sedation often is needed to obtain well-positioned skull or vertebral column radiographs, but is not required to obtain almost lateral or nearly VD views.

When radiographically evaluating the nervous system of a patient, assessment of adjacent skeletal or soft tissue structures also is important,

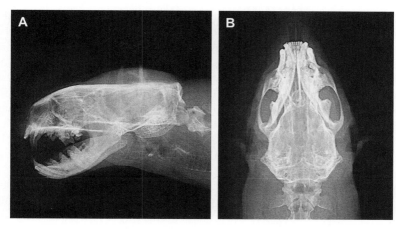

Fig. 1. Lateral (*A*) and ventrodorsal (*B*) radiographic projections of a normal ferret skull. (*Reprinted from* Silverman S, Tell LA. Radiology of rodents, rabbits, and ferrets. St. Louis: Elsevier Saunders; 2005; with permission.)

particularly on skull radiographs. Diseases of the tympanic bulla or the nasal cavities may progress to involve the brain, especially infectious causes (otitis media, sinusitis). Because of the numerous small bones of the skull (especially in birds and small mammals), superimposition of skeletal structures is the most complicating factor in radiographic evaluation. Magnified studies of the skull of small species may enhance the diagnostic value of radiography, but the spatial resolution will be compromised.

Because radiography is based on attenuation of X-rays by bone and soft tissue, the small general mass, and specifically the limited bony mass, of exotic animal species can make interpretation of abnormalities difficult. Additionally, at least 30 to 50% of bone mass must be lost before it is apparent on radiographic studies, so subtle lytic lesions frequently will be missed.

The advantages of radiography are that it is relatively inexpensive, readily available to veterinarians, and good for evaluation of bony production/ lysis and skull and vertebral fractures. The disadvantages include the summation of structures that can make interpretation difficult. Additionally, it is less sensitive than other imaging modalities, so subtle lesions may be missed, and poor positioning may obscure lesions or result in fake ones. Most importantly, radiographic studies do not evaluate neural structures.

Myelography

Myelography is performed after completion of a survey radiographic study of the vertebral column, and it is indicated to evaluate the neural structures. Nonionic iodinated contrast is injected into the subarachnoid space to delineate the spinal cord and identify any compression or distortion of the spinal cord (Fig. 2). If possible, cerebrospinal fluid (CSF) should be collected for analysis, before injection of the radiographic contrast material, to rule out infectious or inflammatory disease. Knowledge of anatomical differences between species is more important for this procedure than any other neurodiagnostic technique. If the subarachnoid space is present, the clinician must know how to access it by means of lumbar or atlanto–occipital puncture. Sampling of the CSF is relatively straightforward in most mammals, but for reptiles, which have no subarachnoid space [8], or birds, which have a glycogen body in the lumbar spinal cord [9] and fusion of the lumbar sacral vertebrae (ie, the synsacrum), CSF collection and myelography are more complicated.

Myelography has been described in small mammals [4,10,11] and in avian [12] and reptile [13,14] species. Myelographic patterns include extradural compression, intradural–extramedullary pattern, and intramedullary pattern, and based on the pattern, the list of potential causes can be modified.

Lesions that would cause an extradural pattern on myelography (Fig. 3) include vertebral fracture/luxation, extradural hemorrhage, disc protrusion or extrusion [11] with spinal cord compression, epidural infection (empyema), vertebral neoplasia, or other extradural neoplasia. Intradural–extramedullary pattern (golf tee appearance) is uncommon and typically is seen with a space-occupying lesion within the subarachnoid space. Intramedullary pattern is present when the lesion is within the spinal cord parenchyma, and this is seen as circumferential attenuation of the contrast columns (Fig. 4 A, B). Possible causes for this pattern include parenchymal infection or inflammation (myelitis), intramedullary hemorrhage, and intramedullary neoplasia.

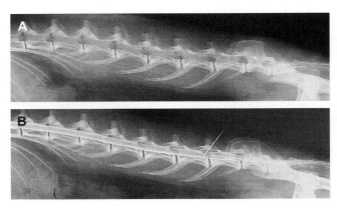

Fig. 2. (*A*) Lateral radiographic projection of the lumbar vertebral column of a domestic rabbit. (*B*) Lateral radiographic projection of a myelogram study of the rabbit lumbar spinal cord. Note the spinal needle placed in the ventral subarachnoid space at L5-6. (*Reprinted from* Silverman S, Tell LA. Radiology of rodents, rabbits, and ferrets. St. Louis: Elsevier Saunders; 2005; with permission.)

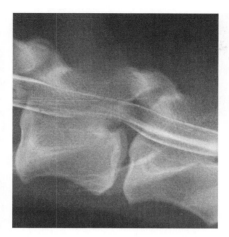

Fig. 3. Lateral radiographic projection of a myelogram study of a dog at the L3-4 vertebral bodies illustrating a ventral extradural compression. Note the dorsal deviation of the contrast columns.

Risks and complications with myelography include the inappropriate introduction of the needle for CSF collection and patient reactions secondary to injection of the contrast. In the lumbar spinal cord, the needle is passed through the parenchyma of the spinal cord to the ventral subarachnoid space, and cisternally, if the needle is advanced too far, the patient may be pithed by direct injury to the brainstem. Transient or permanent neurological damage can result from improper needle placement [12]. In dogs and horses, intrathecal contrast material has been reported to exacerbate neurological deficits and may cause seizures [15–17]. Rarely, in people, aseptic meningitis has been reported secondary to myelography [18].

The advantages of myelography are that it is relatively inexpensive, the entire spinal cord is evaluated relatively quickly, and it delineates extradural lesions well. Disadvantages include that the anatomy of the patient may make myelography difficult or even impossible, it does not permit thorough evaluation of the spinal cord parenchyma, and the potential complications range from transient exacerbation of clinical signs to paralysis and even death [12].

Computed Tomography (CT)

Routine access to CT is becoming increasingly common, and many specialty practices have a CT scanner on-site. Normal CT anatomy of the skull of some exotic animal species has been published [4]. CT uses a radiograph tube and an opposing detector array that are passed around the patient in a 360-degree arc at different intervals. The information obtained at each

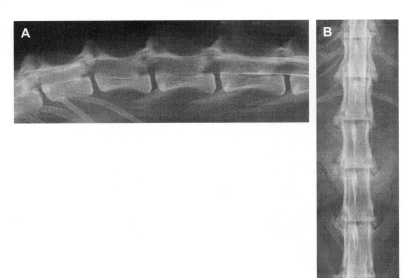

Fig. 4. Lateral (*A*) and ventrodorsal (*B*) radiographic projections of a myelogram study in a cat from T12-L3 vertebral bodies illustrating an intramedullary pattern at L1-2. The circumferential attenuation of the contrast columns indicates an expansile lesion within the parenchyma of the spinal cord.

of these intervals is processed by the computer to form an image of the section (or slice) of tissue at that site. Each slice is a summation of a three-dimensional volume of tissue into a two-dimensional computer image. The thickness of the slice is determined at the time of acquisition. Thinner slices (1 mm) have finer detail than thicker slices (5 to 8 mm), but increase the acquisition time. The appearance of tissue is similar to conventional radiography, although the terminology is different. Air is very hypoattenuating or hypodense (black); soft tissue and fluid are variations of gray. Bone is very hyperattenuating (white), and metallic objects are the most hyperattenuating, producing a dramatic beam-hardening artifact.

CT is uniplanar imaging, and can only obtain cross-sectional images of the tissue passed through the gantry. Software of newer scanners makes it possible to reconstruct the cross-sectional information into different planes, and even into three-dimensional images. CT requires the patient to be immobile for at least 15 to 20 minutes to obtain a diagnostic study, and thus general anesthesia is required for most patients, with the possible exception of some studies of chelonians [19].

CT images are acquired in either soft tissue or bone algorithms, and they can be manipulated to accentuate bone or soft tissue (Figs. 5 and 6). Intravenous iodinated contrast is administered to demonstrate areas with abnormal vascular permeability, such as tumors or regions of inflammation.

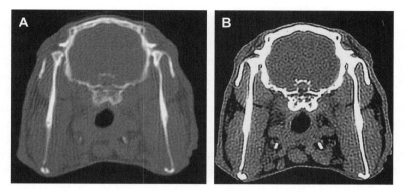

Fig. 5. Transverse computed tomography slices (1 mm thick) of a domestic rabbit skull in bone window (*A*) and soft tissue window (*B*).

Reliable intravenous access is required for postcontrast images, which may be difficult in some exotic species.

Interpretation of CT is easier than conventional radiography, because there is no superimposition of overlying structures. Note how easy it is to appreciate the tympanic bulla cavities in the CT of the ferret in Fig. 6 compared with the radiographs (see Fig. 1). CT provides excellent detail of bone, and evaluating the skull with thin slices will show subtle abnormalities of the fine bones of the nasal passages and frontal sinuses, small fractures of the thick bones of the base of the skull, and abnormalities of the tympanic bulla cavities. Soft tissue evaluation is better with CT than with radiography, but it does not have the same detail as MRI. CT is more sensitive than MRI for acute (<24-hour) hemorrhage, which is hyperattenuating to the surrounding parenchyma.

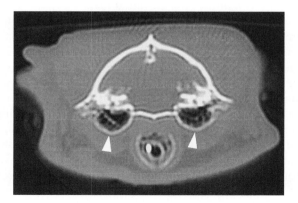

Fig. 6. Transverse CT slices of a normal ferret skull at the level of the tympanic bulla cavities (*arrowheads*). The image is in bone window. (*Reprinted from* Silverman S, Tell LA. Radiology of rodents, rabbits, and ferrets. St. Louis: Elsevier Saunders; 2005; with permission.)

CT after myelography can be very useful, as the contrast within the subarachnoid space highlights the spinal cord. When performing CT of the thoracic or lumbar vertebral column, any nonchelonian patient should be placed in dorsal recumbency, so motion artifact from thoracic wall movement with respiration does not interfere with evaluation of the spinal cord. In addition, interference caused by thoracic wall movement can be minimized using sustained positive-pressure ventilation (breath-holding) during the scan.

The advantages of CT are the removal of superimposed structures, its increasing accessibility, the rapid image acquisition (few minutes), excellent bone detail, and excellent contrast resolution. Because of the increasing accessibility, there are several reports of the clinical use of CT specifically for imaging the skull and vertebral column in exotic animals [20–22]. Disadvantages are that it requires general anesthesia or very heavy sedation; it provides less than ideal soft tissue detail of brain and spinal cord parenchyma, and uniplanar imaging.

Magnetic Resonance Imaging (MRI)

Magnetic resonance technology is very different than radiography and CT. Instead of attenuation of radiographs, MRI uses the molecular composition (particularly the hydrogen atoms, also referred to as protons or spins) of tissue to obtain an image by the principles of nuclear magnetic resonance. The patient is placed within a powerful static magnetic field that aligns the protons in the tissue parallel to the field. Magnet strength is measured in units of Tesla (T), where one T is about 20,000 times the strength of the earth's magnetic field. The transient application of a second electromagnetic pulse (a radiofrequency [RF] pulse) perpendicular to the static field, pushes the protons out of alignment and into a high energy state. When the pulse is stopped, the protons realign with the initial magnetic field, and it is this relaxation of the hydrogen atoms that is detected and used to formulate the image. There are two types of relaxation (T1 and T2 relaxation) that occur to the proton as it returns to equilibrium. The time for T1 and T2 relaxation varies between different tissues. For example, the protons within cortical bone have very different relaxation times than the protons freely moving within CSF.

Similar to CT, magnetic resonance images also are obtained in slices, turning a three-dimensional volume of tissue into a two-dimensional image. One of the advantages of MRI is that images can be obtained in any desired plane without adjusting the patient (multiplanar imaging) (Figs. 7 and 8). Different sequences are obtained, accentuating different aspects of tissues (eg, fluid, fat, edema). Standard imaging sequences are described in subsequent sections, and more technical information about the physics of MRI and other advanced sequences are available to the reader in the article by Seth Wallack, in this issue, as well as through additional references [23–25].

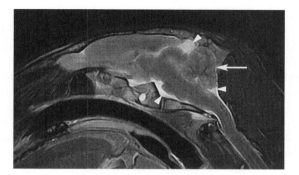

Fig. 7. Sagittal T2-weighted magnetic resonance image of the normal brain of the domestic rabbit. Note hyperintense cerebrospinal fluid (*arrowheads*) surrounding the brainstem and cerebellum (*arrow*). Image was obtained with a 1.5 T magnet with 3 mm slice thickness.

Common imaging sequences

T1-weighted images are obtained pre- and post-contrast. Fluid, like CSF, is hypointense (blacker) compared with gray matter (Fig. 8A). Intravenous gadolinium (a rare earth element) is administered to obtain post-contrast images, and this requires intravenous access. Similar to CT, contrast enhancement is seen with inflammation, infection, and some neoplasia, indicating increased vascular permeability or an abnormal blood–brain or blood–spinal cord barrier (Fig. 9).

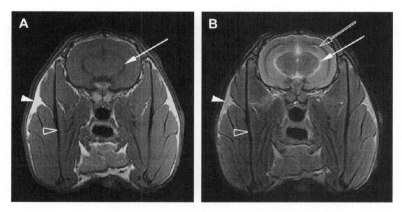

Fig. 8. Transverse T1-weighted (*A*) and T2-weighted (*B*) magnetic resonance images of the normal brain of a domestic rabbit. Note the different intensity of cerebrospinal fluid surrounding the brain (*closed arrows*)—hypointense on the T1-weighted image (*A*), and hyperintense on the T2-weighted image (*B*). Subcutaneous fat is hyperintense on both images (*closed arrowhead*), and the cortical bone of the mandible (*open arrowhead*) is hypointense on both images. The difference between the white matter (*open arrow*) and the adjacent gray matter in the cerebral cortex is appreciated readily on the T2-weighted image (*B*). Images were obtained with a 1.5 T magnet, and slice thickness is 3 mm.

On T2-weighted images, fluid (CSF and edema) appears hyperintense (whiter) when compared with gray matter (see Fig. 7 and Fig. 8B). The gray and white matter interface is more apparent on T2 weighted images than T1 images.

Fluid attenuated inversion recovery (FLAIR) images are essentially T2-weighted images in which free fluid (CSF) is "blacked out", making parenchymal fluid (edema) more apparent (Fig. 10).

Proton density (PD) images demonstrate fluid and tissue somewhere between T1 and T2, and delineate the gray and white matter interface well.

Cortical bone and air are very hypointense, and fat is very hyperintense on all standard imaging sequences. Note the signal intensity of bone and subcutaneous fat in Figs. 7–9.

Additional special sequences to emphasize or suppress the signals from different tissues are obtained at the discretion of the clinician based on clinical indication (eg, fat saturation [suppresses signal from fat], gradient echo [emphasizes inhomogeneities in the magnetic field], diffusion- and perfusion-weighted imaging [to evaluate perfusion to tissue], among others). These additional sequences can give the clinician valuable information about the patient's disease process, but prolong the MRI scanning time.

MRI has revolutionized diagnostic evaluation of the brain and spinal cord of the canine and feline species. It is certainly the preferred method for imaging the soft tissue of the brain, and often for imaging the spinal cord. There are publications describing normal magnetic resonance anatomy [26] and magnetic resonance appearance of numerous different pathological processes of the dog and cat, but there are very few reports

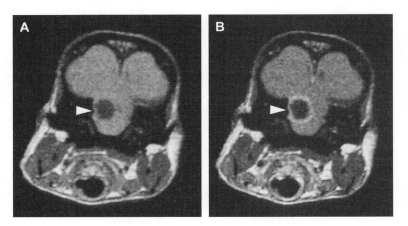

Fig. 9. Transverse T1-weighted pre-contrast (*A*) and post-contrast (*B*) magnetic resonance images at the level of the pons of a Chinese crested goose. There is a hypointense lesion in the brainstem that enhances in a ring pattern after intravenous administration of gadolinium contrast (*arrowheads*). Histopathology of the lesion diagnosed a mycobacterial abscess. Images were obtained with a 0.5 T magnet and slice thickness is 4 mm.

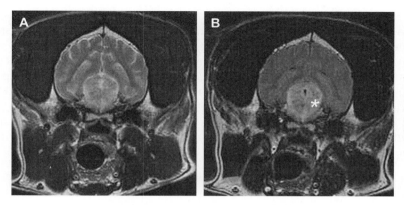

Fig. 10. Transverse T2-weighted (*A*) and fluid-attenuated inversion recovery (*B*) magnetic resonance images at the level of the midbrain of a dog presenting for progressive obtundation. When the signal from the CSF is nulled, the persistent hyperintensity within the midbrain is very apparent (*asterisk*), suggestive of parenchymal edema.

of clinical MRI of the CNS of exotic animal species in the veterinary literature [21,27–30]. Several factors likely are involved in the currently limited use of MRI, including availability, cost, length of scan time, and patient size.

Availability

The specialized equipment and shielding needed to house a magnetic resonance magnet are very expensive, thus MRI is typically available only at specialty referral centers or institutions. Very high field magnets (>4.0 T) produce excellent images of small patients, but are used almost exclusively for research [31–35].

Cost

Cost of scanning varies between locations, but typically ranges between $800 and $1800, excluding cost of anesthesia.

Length of scan time

Depending on the scanning protocols, the number of sequences obtained, and whether contrast is given, MRI scan time can range from 40 to 60 minutes for standard imaging sequences (T1 pre- and post-contrast in transverse and sagittal planes, T2, plus or minus FLAIR), to much longer if additional sequences are done. Patients must be completely still for these scans, necessitating general anesthesia. The limited monitoring in the magnetic resonance gantry increases the risk of prolonged anesthesia, especially in small patients that rapidly lose body heat.

Some imaging protocols in veterinary medicine rely heavily on very rapid imaging sequences, such as HASTE (half acquisition single-shot turbo spin echo), where slices are acquired within 2 to 3 seconds. The advantage of the HASTE sequence is the short scan time. The signal-to-noise ratio (SNR) is lower than with conventional sequences, however, and this can make interpretation difficult. There are methods of improving the SNR, but they have their own limitations (see "Improving signal-to-noise ratio in small patients").

Patient size

Magnetic resonance is based on excitation of a volume of tissue and recording the echo from that tissue. If the excited volume of tissue is small, the echo is small, and the image resolution is poor. Typically, 3- to 5 mm slices of tissue are excited, but for a patient whose brain is only 3- to 4 cm long or whose spinal cord is less than 1 cm wide, the loss of anatomical detail through averaging thick slices will complicate interpretation of the image, and some lesions may be missed. Unlike CT, where obtaining thin slices can improve detail, in MRI, thin slices of tissue have less volume and can result in poor SNR. There are several ways to improve the SNR when imaging a small patient. Adjustments in either the hardware or the software can make a big difference, but facilities and patient welfare are ultimately limiting factors.

Because of the strong magnetic field, specialized anesthesia equipment without ferrous or metal parts must be used. Most of this equipment is designed for larger patients, and cannot be adequately adapted for very small patients with small tidal volumes.

Improving signal-to-noise ratio in small patients

Increased magnet strength

Increased field strength will increase SNR. High-field magnets (>4 T) produce exquisitely detailed images on small patients, but are less available to clinicians than 0.5 to 1.5 T magnets. Compare the grainy image quality of Fig. 9, obtained with a 0.5 T magnet, with the image quality of Fig. 8, obtained with a 1.5 T magnet.

Coil type

The closer the receiver coils can get to the tissue imaged, the better the SNR. Different types of coils will permit this. Commonly used coils for MRI in veterinary medicine are human knee coils, other extremity coils, and quadrature coils, among others.

Increased number of excitations

Increasing the number of times the slice of tissue is excited and the signal recorded will increase the SNR. Number of excitations (NEX) is related directly to scan time, but not directly to SNR. To double the SNR solely by manipulation of the NEX, the NEX (and therefore the scan and anesthesia time) would have to be quadrupled [36].

Increased slice thickness

Slice thickness is directly related to SNR, so doubling the slice thickness will double the SNR [24,36]. The concerns with loss of anatomical detail from acquiring thick slices in very small patients have been discussed previously, so the clinician and MRI technologist must reach a balance between imaging a large enough volume of tissue to produce a sufficient echo and a slice thin enough to demonstrate anatomy.

The advantages of MRI are that it provides excellent soft tissue and anatomical detail, the different sequences can evaluate different aspects of soft tissue, and it permits multiplanar imaging. Disadvantages include the expense, limited availability, the long scanning time, and, for small exotic animal species, the difficulties of imaging small patients.

Summary

Imaging the CNS of companion exotic veterinary patients frequently is required to accurately diagnose and subsequently treat their diseases. Based on the patient's neuroanatomical localization and the knowledge of the perks and pitfalls of the different imaging modalities, the clinician can choose the most appropriate modality to evaluate the brain or spinal cord. Because the availability and use of advanced imaging are increasing in veterinary medicine, it is important for exotic animal clinicians to know how to maximize the diagnostic yield of CT and MRI for their patients.

Acknowledgments

The author thanks Richard Larson and Jason Peters, for acquisition of images, John Doval for assistance with figures, and Eric Johnson, DVM, Diplomate ACVR, for technical consultation.

References

[1] Rubel G, Isenbugel E, Wolvekamp P. Atlas of diagnostic radiology of exotic pets. Philadelphia: W.B. Saunders; 1991.
[2] Paul-Murphy J, Koblik PD, Stein G, et al. Psittacine skull radiography. Veterinary Radiology 1990;31:218–24.
[3] Redrobe S. Imaging techniques in small mammals. Seminars in Avian and Exotic Pet Medicine 2001;10:187–97.
[4] Silverman S, Tell LA. Radiology of rodents, rabbits, and ferrets. St. Louis (MO): Elsevier Saunders; 2005.

[5] Ramsay E, Daniel GB, Tryon BW, et al. Osteomyelitis associted with *Salmonella enterica* ss. *arizonae* in a colony of Ridgenose rattlesnakes (*Crotalus willardi*). J Zoo Wildl Med 2002;33: 301–10.

[6] Isaza R, Garner M, Jacobson E. Proliferative osteoarthritis and osteoarthrosis in 15 snakes. J Zoo Wildl Med 2000;31:20–7.

[7] Rhody J, Schiller CA. Spinal osteosarcoma in a hedgehog with pedal self-mutilation. Vet Clin North Am Exot Anim Pract 2006;9:625–31.

[8] Keeble E. Neurology. In: Girling S, Raiti P, editors. BSAVA manual of reptiles. 2nd edition. Gloucester (UK): British Small Animal Veterinary Association; 2004. p. 273–88.

[9] King A. Birds—their structure and function. 2nd edition. London: Bailliere Tindall; 1984.

[10] Antinoff N. Musculoskeletal and neurologic diseases. In: Quesenberry KECJ, editor. Ferrets, rabbits, and rodents: clinical medicine and surgery. 2nd edition. Philadelphia: Saunders; 1997. p. 115–20.

[11] Morera N, Mascort J. Intervertebral disc prolapse in a ferret. Vet Clin North Am Exot Anim Pract 2006;9:667–71.

[12] Harr K, Kollias GV, Rendano V, et al. A myelographic technique for avian species. Vet Radiol Ultrasound 1997;38:187–92.

[13] Schumacher J, Toal RL. Advanced radiography and ultrasonography in reptiles. Seminars in Avian and Exotic Pet Medicine 2001;10:162–8.

[14] Divers S, Lawton MPC. Spinal osteomyelitis in a green iguana,*Iguana iguana*: cerebrospinal fluid and myelogram diagnosis. Reno (NV): Association of Reptilian and Amphibian Veterinarians; 2000. p. 77.

[15] Barone G, Zeimer LS, Shofer FS, et al. Risk factors associated with development of seizures after use of iohexol for myelography in dogs: 182 cases (1998). J Am Vet Med Assoc 2002; 220:1499–502.

[16] Lewis D, Hosgood G. Complications associated with the use of iohexol for myelography of the cervical vertebral column in dogs: 66 cases (1988–1990). J Am Vet Med Assoc 1992;200: 1381–4.

[17] Widmer W, Blevins WE, Jakovijevic S, et al. A prospective clinical trial comparing metrizamide and iohexol for equine myelography. Vet Radiol Ultrasound 1998;39:106–9.

[18] Bender A, Elstner M, Paul R, et al. Severe symptomatic aseptic chemical meningitis following myelography—the role of procalcitonin. Neurology 2004;63:1311–3.

[19] Gumpenberger M. Computed tomography (CT) in chelonians. Reno (NV): Association of Reptilian and Amphibian Veterinarians; 2002. p. 41–3.

[20] de Voe R, Pack L, Greenacre CB. Radiographic and CT imaging of a skull associated osteoma in a ferret. Vet Radiol Ultrasound 2002;43:346–8.

[21] Spaulding K, Loomis MR. Principles and applications of computed tomography and magnetic resonance imaging in zoo and wildlife medicine. In: Fowler M, Miller RE, editors. Zoo & wildlife animal medicine. 4th edition. Philadelphia: W.B. Saunders; 1999. p. 83–8.

[22] Bartels T, Krautwald-Junghanns M-E, Portmann S, et al. The use of conventional radiography and computer-assisted tomography as instruments for demonstration of gross pathological lesions in the cranium and cerebrum in the crested breed of the domestic duck (*Anas platyrhynchos* f. dom.). Avian Pathol 2000;29:101–8.

[23] Thomson C, Kornegay JN, Burn RA, et al. Magnetic resonance imaging—a general overview of principles and examples in veterinary neurodiagnostics. Vet Radiol Ultrasound 1993;34:2–17.

[24] Young IR, Bydder GM. Contrast development and manipulation in MR imaging. In: Atlas S, editor. Magnetic resonance imaging of the brain and spine. 3rd edition. Philadelphia: Lippincott Williams & Wilkins; 2002. p. 33–58.

[25] Moseley M, Saswyer-Glover A, Kucharczyk J. Magnetic resonance imaging principles and techniques. In: Latchaw R, Kucharczyk J, Moseley ME, editors. Imaging of the nervous system diagnostic and therapeutic applications. Philadephia: Elsevier Mosby; 2005. p. 3–31.

[26] Assheuer J, Sager M. MRI and CT atlas of the dog. Oxford: Blackwell Science; 1997.

[27] Romagnano A, Shiroma JT, Heard DJ, et al. Magnetic resonance imaging of the brain and coelomic cavity of the domestic pigeon (*Columba livia domestica*). Vet Radiol Ultrasound 1996;37:431–40.

[28] Morgan R, Donnell RL, Daniel GB. Magnetic resonance imaging of the normal eye and orbit of a screech owl (otus asio). Vet Radiol Ultrasound 1994;35:362–7.

[29] Bartels T, Brinkmeier J, Portmann S, et al. Magnetic resonance imaging of intracranial tissue accumulations in domestic ducks (*Anas platyrhynchos* f. dom.) with feather crests. Vet Radiol Ultrasound 2001;42:254–8.

[30] Pye G, Bennet RA, Roberts GD, et al. Thoracic vertebral chordoma in a domestic ferret (*Mustela putorius furo*). J Zoo Wildl Med 2000;31:107–11.

[31] Mirrashed F, Sharp JC, Cheung I, et al. High-resolution imaging at 3T and 7T with multiring local volume coils. MAGMA 2004;16:167–73.

[32] Wang L-C, Jung S-M, Chen C-C, et al. Pathological changes in the brains of rabbits experimentally infected with *Angiostrongylus cantonensis* after albendazole treatment: histopathological and magnetic resonance imaging studies. J Antimicrob Chemother 2006;57:294–300.

[33] Neal J, Takahashi M, Silva M, et al. Insights into the gyrification of developing ferret brain by magnetic resonance imaging. J Anat 2007;210:66–77.

[34] Van Meir V, Pavlova D, Verhoye M, et al. In vivo MR imaging of the seasonal volumetric and functional plasticity of song control nuclei in relation to song output in a female songbird. Neuroimage 2006;31:981–92.

[35] Anderson C, Kabalka GW, Layne DG, et al. Noninvasive high-field MRI brain imaging of the garter snake (*Thamnophis sirtalis*). Copeia 2000;1:265–9.

[36] Runge V, Nitz WR, Schmeets SH, et al. The physics of clinical MR taught through images. New York: Thieme Medical Publishers; 2005.

VETERINARY
CLINICS
Exotic Animal Practice

ELSEVIER
SAUNDERS

Vet Clin Exot Anim 10 (2007) 909–925

Basic Magnetic Resonance Imaging Principles Used for Evaluating Animal Patients with Neurologic Disease

Seth Wallack, DVM, DACVR

Veterinary Imaging Center of San Diego, Inc. and DVMinsight-premier teleradiology,
San Diego, CA, USA

MRI use in veterinary medicine, and in particular in exotic animals, is growing in popularity, because it provides excellent anatomic and pathologic detail. Performing a useful MRI study, however, depends on the user choosing the correct pulse sequences. Without an understanding of MRI pulse sequences, it is difficult to perform and interpret a study. A solid foundation of MRI principles will be far more useful for image interpretation than just a case-by-case review showing pathology, because even cases of the same disease may have a dissimilar appearance.

MRI physics

MRI works by aligning hydrogen protons. Each proton spins on an axis. The magnetic field generated within the bore of the MRI aligns those spins in a parallel and antiparallel arrangement along the external magnetic field called Bo and results in longitudinal magnetization (Fig. 1) [1]. The nuclei, however, do not spin perfectly but instead have a wobble or precession. The precession frequency is a constant for each atom within a specific magnetic field, and is mathematically determined by the Larmor equation [2]. Hydrogen atoms have a precessional frequency of 42.57 MHz/T [3]. This wobble is synchronized when a radiofrequency (RF) is applied. The synchronized wobble results in transverse magnetization. Another way to conceptualize the wobble is to think of each nucleus as a merry-go-round with one child (electron) somewhere along the edge. Now picture a field of 100 merry-go-rounds with one child on each one. The Bo magnetic field results in

E-mail address: seth@vicsd.com

1094-9194/07/$ - see front matter © 2007 Elsevier Inc. All rights reserved.
doi:10.1016/j.cvex.2007.04.005   *vetexotic.theclinics.com*

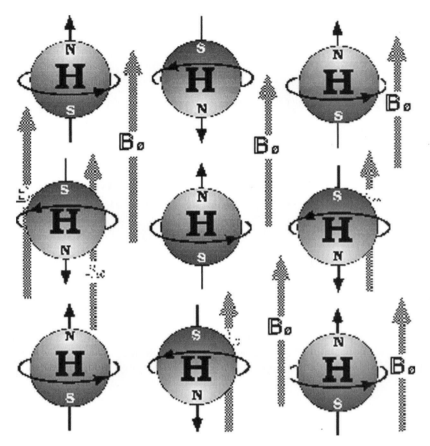

Fig. 1. Hydrogen atoms aligned in the parallel and antiparallel direction along the external magnetic field termed Bo. (*Courtesy of* Simply Physics, Baltimore, MD; with permission. Available at: www.simplyphysics.com. Accessed December 18, 2006.)

most of the merry-go-rounds pointing in the same location. When the specific RF pulse is applied to the nuclei, it not only causes the synchronized wobble, but also shifts the alignment of the nuclei out of the parallel/antiparallel alignment and to a new direction. This is termed the flip angle and decreases the longitudinal magnetization built by Bo.

When the RF pulse is stopped, the longitudinal magnetization rebuilds, because the nuclei realign with Bo. At the same time, the unified wobbling nuclei start to go out of unison (dephase), and the transverse magnetization is lost. The increase in longitudinal magnetization and decrease in transverse magnetization are detected by the coils as a signal, and through computer processing, a magnetic resonance image is created. The regain of longitudinal relaxation is termed T1 (Fig. 2), and the decrease in transverse magnetization is T2* (* is pronounced star) and T2 (Fig. 3). The T2* is different

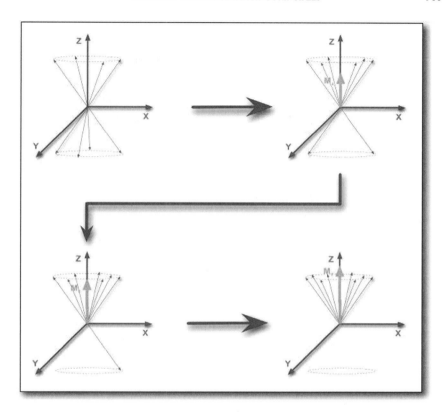

Fig. 2. Rebuilding of longitudinal signal that correlates to T1 weighting for MRI. The larger arrow along the Z axis indicates the overall magnetization vector. This longitudinal magnetization rebuilds inline with the external magnetic field (Bo) once the radiofrequency pulse is stopped.

from the T2, because it identifies focal loss of unified precession due to regional tissue magnetic field inhomogeneities caused by the presence of such things as metal, bone, or air.

Tissue differences in T1, T2, and T2* properties and proton density are identified by varying the time to repetition (TR) and time to echo (TE) intervals [4]. TR is the time between the application of two separate RF excitation sequences [5,6]. TE is the time between the RF excitation and the peak of the detected echo [5,6]. Both TR and TE affect MRI contrast. Short TR intervals and long TE intervals are used to enhance the difference in longitudinal and transverse relaxation, respectively, between fat and water. Long TR and short TE intervals identify the difference in proton density between tissue types, with tissues with a higher proton density having a higher signal intensity (Table 1).

Although MRI is considered safe, and no ionizing radiation is used, the concept of specific absorption rate (SAR) is applied to MRI [7]. The RF

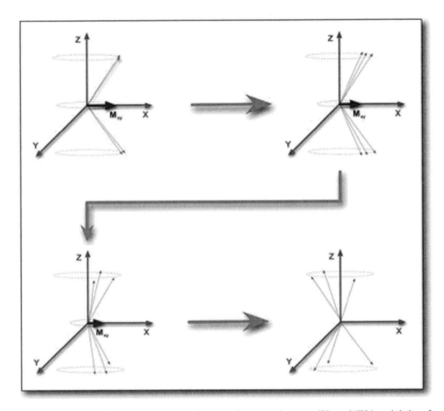

Fig. 3. Relaxation of transverse magnetization that correlates to T2 and T2* weighting for MRI. The larger arrow along the X axis indicates the overall magnetization vector before stopping the radiofrequency pulse. Notice how this arrow becomes smaller as the nuclei dephase resulting in a loss of signal.

pulse used to flip the magnetization vector into the transverse plane deposits energy into the patient. The SAR is a measurement in watts that quantifies the rate at which RF energy is dissipated in tissue. The SAR relates directly to the field strength, flip angle, and TR frequency and if the field strength or flip angle is doubled, then the SAR increases fourfold. If the TR frequency is doubled, then the SAR also is doubled.

Table 1
Effect of time to repetition and time to echo on MRI contrast

Imaging technique	Time to repetition	Time to echo
T1 weighting	Short	Short
T2 weighting	Long	Long
Proton density weighting	Long	Short

Tissue weighting

Altering TR and TE intervals is used to emphasize a particular tissue type. This selection of TR and TE intervals is termed image weighting.

T1 weighting

T1 weighting uses a short TR and short TE. T1 weighted images depict anatomy and are used when gadolinium contrast is administered (Figs. 4 and 5).

T2 weighting

T2 weighting uses a long TR and a long TE. T2 weighted images depict fluid accumulations and edema. Because most diseased tissues have a high water content, they are depicted best on this study and will be bright (hyperintense) (Figs. 6 and 7).

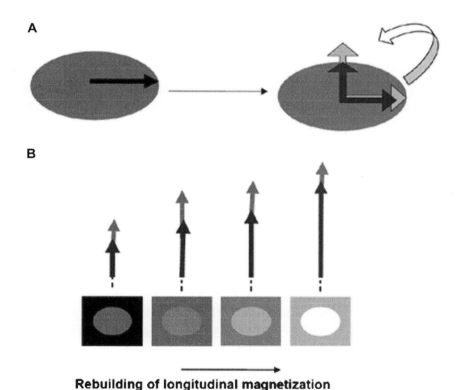

Rebuilding of longitudinal magnetization

Fig. 4. Magnetic resonance T1 weighted image with contrast. (*A*) Rebuilding of longitudinal magnetization. (*B*) difference in T1 contrast as longitudinal magnetization rebuilds.

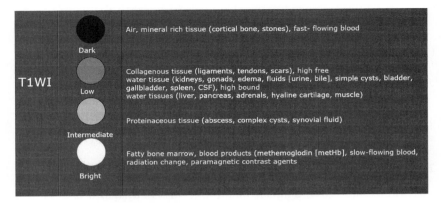

Fig. 5. Diagram shows the signal intensity of various tissues at T1 weighted MRI. Note, however, that the signal characteristics of proteinaceous tissues vary according to the amount of protein content. Tissues with high concentrations of protein may have high signal intensity on T1 weighted images (*T1WI*). *Abbreviation:* CSF, cerebrospinal fluid. (*From* Bitar R, Leung G, Perng R, et al. MR pulse sequences: what every radiologist wants to know but is afraid to ask. RadioGraphics 2006;26:513–37; with permission.)

Pulse sequences

The pulse sequence is the combination of the magnetic gradients and TR pulses used in magnetic resonance image acquisition. There are two fundamental types of magnetic resonance pulse sequences, spin echo (SE) and gradient recall echo (GRE) (Tables 2 and 3). GE Healthcare (Milwaukee, Wisconsin), Siemens (New York, New York), and Philips (Bothell, Washington) have proprietary trade names for similar pulse sequences. Table 4 lists the common and trade names for the more common pulse sequences used.

Spin echo

A 90-degree RF pulse flips the magnetic vector into the transverse plane [8]. As the tissue goes through T1, T2, and T2* relaxation, the transverse magnetization gradually is lost. To rebuild the magnetization, a second 180-degree pulse is applied, at a time equal to one-half of the TE. Analogous would be 10 runners starting out together but moving at different speeds. At exactly half way into the race, all the runners would turn around and run back to the start. If the runners maintained a steady pace they should all return back to the starting line at exactly the same moment. At the point of TE, the nuclei should be spinning in phase and the strongest echo acquired. Conventional SE pulses are long and have been replaced with fast or turbo SE sequences.

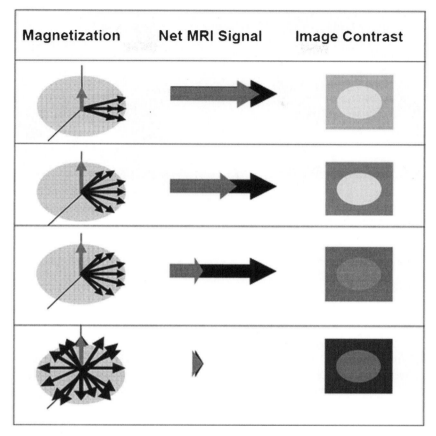

Fig. 6. T2 contrast. (*Left column*) Transverse magnetization is lost from top to bottom. (*Center column*) Nuclear magnetic resonance (NMR) signal decreases as transverse magnetization is lost. (*Right column*) Difference in T2 contrast as transverse magnetization is lost.

Fast or turbo spin echo

A single 90-degree pulse is applied after which several 180-degree re-phrasing pulses are applied at one-half of each TE [9]. The collection of echoes is referred to as an echo train length.

Inversion recovery

This sequence is used to null the signal from a specific tissue type. This is accomplished by applying an initial 180-degree pulse and then when that specific tissue passes through the null point for that tissue, the conventional 90-degree pulse is applied. The interval between the initial 180-degree pulse and the 90-degree pulse is the inversion time (TI). The two standard

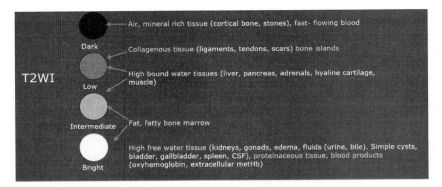

Fig. 7. Diagram shows the signal intensity of various tissues at T2 weighted MRI. However, note, however that the signal characteristics of proteinaceous tissues vary according to the amount of protein content: Tissues with high concentrations of protein may have low signal intensity on T2-weighted images (T2W1). *Abbreviation:* CSF, cerebrospinal fluid. (*From* Bitar R, Leung G, Perng R, et al. MR pulse sequences: what every radiologist wants to know but is afraid to ask. RadioGraphics 2006;26:513–37; with permission.)

inversion recovery sequences are STIR (short T1 inversion-recovery) and FLAIR (fluid-attenuated inversion-recovery).

Short T1 inversion-recovery

This sequence is used to null the fat signal [10]. The 90-degree pulse is applied approximately 140 ms (null point for fat) after the initial 180-degree pulse. STIR sequences are used for bone marrow edema, which can be found with fractures (Fig. 8).

Fluid-attenuated inversion-recovery

This sequence is used to null the signal from free water and particularly cerebrospinal fluid (CSF) [11]. FLAIR sequences are used to differentiate free fluid from parenchymal edema or periventricular lesions (Figs. 9 and 10).

Gradient recall echo

In the gradient recall echo (GRE) sequence, the applied RF pulse only partly flips the magnetization vector (<90 degrees), whereas in SE, a 90-

Table 2
Comparison between spin echo and gradient recall echo sequences from MRI

Criterion	Spin echo	Gradient recall echo
Rephasing mechanism	Radiofrequency pulse	Variation of gradients
Flip angle	90° only	Variable
Efficiency at reducing magnetic inhomogeneity	Very efficient (true T2 weighting)	Not very efficient (T2* weighting)
Acquisition time	Long (slow sequences)	Short (fast sequences)

Table 3

Typical time to repetition and time to echo values for spin echo and gradient recall echo sequences from MRI

Sequence	Time to repetition		Time to echo	
	Short	Long	Short	Long
Spin echo	250–700	> 2000	10–25	> 60
Gradient recall echo	< 50	> 100	1–5	> 10

Values are given in milliseconds

degree pulse is used [12]. Gradients, as opposed to RF pulses, then are used to rephrase the GRE sequences. GRE sequences are very sensitive to magnetic field inhomogeneity between tissues. This quality is used in GRE sequences to detect hemorrhage, because the iron associated with hemorrhage causes field inhomogeneity and enhances T2* signal decay [13]. Discovered in the early 1990s and being used more commonly in research the quantity of deoxyhemoglobin, which also causes magnetic inhomogeneity, GRE has been used in the study of brain function [14]. GRE studies use a short TR, keeping the nuclei in a steady state of precession, making T2* the predominant determination of image contrast (see Tables 2 and 3).

Gradient recall echo sequences can be refocused fully, partially refocused, or spoiled

Partially refocused or coherent gradient recall echo

A gradient called a rewind gradient is used to rephrase the T2* magnetization, preserving the T2* effects [15,16]. This sequence provides T2 weighting. These sequences are used in magnetic resonance angiography.

Fully refocused gradient recall echo

This sequence is like the partially refocused, but all the gradients are refocused. Additionally, the RF pulse phase is alternated between 0 and 180 degrees. This alternation results in an improved signal. These sequences use a short TR because of their inhomogenity susceptibility, but they provide images with a high signal-to-noise ratio. The rapid acquisition time makes this sequence useful in cardiac imaging and interventional magnetic resonance.

Partially of fully refocused GRE sequences are termed GRASS by GE Healthcare, FISP by Siemens, and FFE by Philips.

Spoiled gradient recall echo

This sequence uses a spoiler RF pulse or gradient to eliminate remaining transverse magnetization [17]. Unspoiled GRE sequences have a T2

Table 4
Common and trade names used for spin echo, inversion-recovery sequences, and gradient recall echo sequences from MRI

Common and trade names for spin echo sequences used by major vendors			
Pulse sequence	GE Healthcare	Siemens Medical Solutions	Philips Medical Systems
Single-echo Spin echo (SE)	SE	Single SE	SE, modified SE
Multiple-echo SE	Multiecho multiplanar (MEMP), variable echo multiplanar (VEMP)	SE double echo	Multiple SE (MSE)
Echo-train SE (SSFSE)	Fast SE (FSE), single-shot fast SE, TurboSE (TSE) half Fourier acquisition turbo SE (HASTE)	TSE, ultrafast SE (UFSE)	

Inversion recovery (IR) sequences used by major vendors			
Pulse sequence	GE Healthcare	Siemens Medical Solutions	Philips Medical Systems
Standard IR	Multiplanar inversion recovery (MPIR)	IR	IR
Echo-train IR	Fast multiplanar IR (FMPIR)	TurboIR	IR-turboSE
Short T1 IR	STIR	STIR	Spectrally selective IR (SPIR)
Note: STIR, short inversion time IR.			

Gradient recall echo sequences used by major vendors			
Pulse sequence	GE Healthcare	Siemens Medical Solutions	Philips Medical Systems
Refocused, after excitation	Gradient-recalled acquisition in the steady state (GRASS), fast GRASS, multiplanar GRASS (FMPGR)	Fast imaging with steady-state precession (FISP)	Fast field echo (FFE)
Spoiled (incoherent)	Spoiled GRASS (SPGR), fast spoiled GRASS (FSPGR), multiplanar spoiled GRASS (MPSPGR), fast multiplanar spoiled GRASS (FMPSPGR)	Fast low-angle shot (FLASH)	T1-weighted contrast-enhanced FFE (T1 CE-FFE)
Refocused, pre-exicitation	SSFP	Reversed FISP (PSIF)	T2-weighted contrast-enhanced FFE (T2 CE-FFE)
Magnetization prepared	IR-prepared fast GRASS	Turbo FLASH, magnetization-prepared rapid acquisition gradient echo (MP-RAGE)	Turbo field echo (TFE)

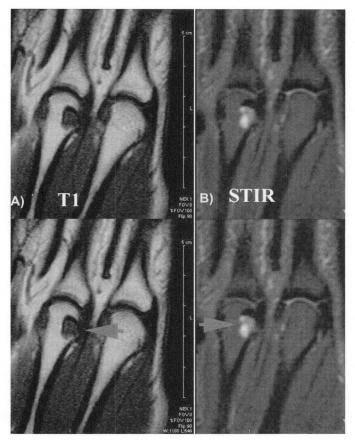

Fig. 8. Short T1 inversion-recovery (STIR) magnetic resonance images of a human hand. (*A*) Normal T1 weighted (*B*) STIR (fat suppressed image). The arrow is pointing to an erosion in the radial side of the third metacarpal. STIR images confirm the presence of this erosion. Bright STIR signal suggests its subacute nature. (*Courtesy of* Boca Radiology Group, Boca Raton, Florida; with permission.)

weighting, while spoiled GRE sequences have a T1 weighting, because they evaluate rebuilding of the longitudinal magnetization. This sequence is useful in contrast magnetic resonance.

Spoiled GRE sequences are termed spoiled GRASS by GE, FLASH by Siemens, and T1-weighted FFE by Philips (see Table 4).

Echo planar imaging

This sequence uses a single TR echo train to obtain data for the entire image slice. This sequence is used when a short acquisition time is essential [18]. Both SE and GRE sequences can be used in echo planar imaging. Echo planar SE imaging provides high tissue contrast, and it is used for cerebral

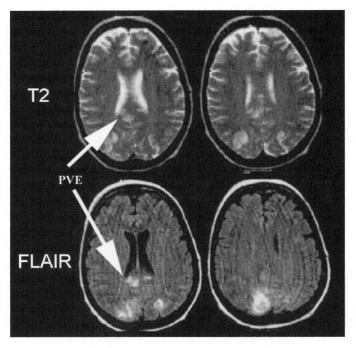

Fig. 9. Magnetic resonance coronal images of the human brain. T2 weighted versus fluid-attenuated inversion-recovery (FLAIR) images. T2 images are on top and FLAIR on bottom. The
FLAIR images null the signal from cerebral spinal fluid (CSF) but keep the non-CSF fluid signal bright, making identification of edematous regions easier. This technique is particularly
important with periventricular edema, which is present in these images (*arrows*). *Abbreviation:*
PVE, periventricular edema.

diffusion weighted imaging. Echo planar imaging is highly vulnerable to
magnetic susceptibility effects.

Diffusion weighted imaging

This sequence enables distinguishing between unrestricted and restricted
diffusion of protons [19]. Restricted proton diffusion is present in cases of
acute stroke. Diffusion weighted imaging uses either echo planar or a fast
GRE sequence. Two equal gradients are applied, and if there is restricted
proton flow (acute stroke) and no proton movement occurs between the opposite pulses, then high signal intensity is present. If normal proton movement is present, then the signal intensity is decreased. This low versus
high signal allows differentiation of regions affected by acute stroke. Typically diffusion weighted imaging is obtained in conjunction with T2
weighted images, and it is used in combination to determine apparent diffusion coefficient (ADC) mapping. Hypointense regions on ADC maps indicate regions of restricted diffusion (acute stroke), and hyperintense regions
correspond to areas of unrestricted diffusion.

Occasionally, a high signal on diffusion-weighted imaging can be caused by T2 effects termed T2 shine-through. In this instance, the ADC map used in conjunction with diffusion weighted images allows determination of the age of a stroke. Dark areas on the combined diffuse weighted and ADC images indicate areas of acute stroke, while the opposite is true about regions of old stroke (Fig. 10).

Magnetic resonance angiography

Time-of-flight (TOF), phase contrast imaging, contrast-enhanced magnetic resonance angiography, and multiple overlapping thin-slab acquisitions are sequences used for magnetic resonance angiography (Fig. 11).

Time-of-flight and multiple overlapping thin-slab acquisition

In these sequences, multiple RF pulses are applied with short TRs saturating the stationary tissue in an imaging slab [20,21]. Inflowing blood is unaffected by the tissue saturation, and the inflowing blood appears hyperintense compared with the stationary tissue. TOF imaging can be acquired in two-dimensional sections or in larger three-dimensional volumes. Multiple overlapping thin-slab acquisition (MOTSA) is a hybrid of two- and three-dimensional TOF imaging, but each slab is thinner than the typical three-dimensional TOF slab.

Phase contrast imaging

This sequence provides information about the flow direction and velocity [22]. This sequence requires two measurements, with each measurement

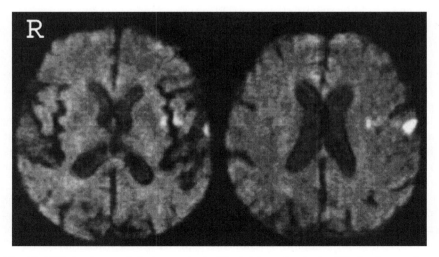

Fig. 10. Diffusion image of the human brain. The bright region in the diffusion images show acute infarction in the left peri-sylvian region.

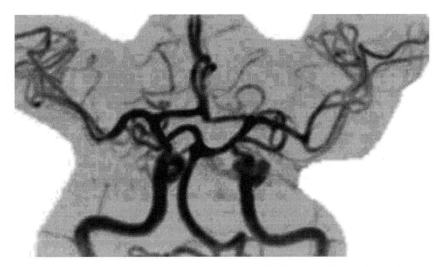

Fig. 11. Magnetic resonance angiography of the circle of Willis in the human brain. This type of imaging study provides a noninvasive evaluation of intracranial vessels without injections and can assess atherosclerosis and aneurysms reliably in people.

sensitized to flow in opposing directions. The measurements are subtracted, resulting in no signal from stationary tissue and signal only from flowing blood.

Contrast-enhanced magnetic resonance angiography

This sequence uses intravenous contrast shortening the T1 of blood, resulting in high signal intensity of T1-weighted images [23].

Fat suppression

Typically fat has a high signal intensity on T1 weighted images. Sometimes, however, it is desirable to null the high signal intensity from fat to improve visualization of the nonfat tissues. In these situations, various fat saturation or nullification methods can be used. Fat saturation may be obtained by applying an RF pulse at the beginning of a sequence followed by a spoiler gradient that shifts the net magnetization vector of fat so that fat has no longitudinal magnetization at the time of image acquisition [24]. This results in no signal from fat. Fat saturation techniques are used clinically for liposarcomas and bone marrow to null the fat signal.

The second method for fat saturation is the use of inversion-recovery pulse or STIR to null fat signal [10]. This inversion pulse is used when the net magnetization vector of fat passes the null point. At this null point, there is little to no longitudinal magnetization present, and when the 90-degree RF pulse is applied at this null point, the transverse magnetization of fat is insignificant, resulting in no signal generated from fat (see Fig. 8).

The third method of fat saturation involves the process of only exciting tissues containing water [25]. Since fat is hydrophobic there is no transverse magnetization generated in fat and therefore no signal generated. The spectral-spatial RF pulse is one example of this water excitation technique.

In-phase and out-of-phase imaging

This technique is used to identify microscopic fat. Identification of microscopic fat is important in differentiating some tumor types in people such as adrenal adenomas versus carcinomas. This technique uses the fact that hydrogen molecules precess at different rates depending on their surrounding environment. Fat and water are imaged with their hydrogen nuclei spinning in phase and out of phase with each other. If microscopic fat is present, the fat signal is nulled on the out-of-phase images [26]. This technique frequently uses a spoiled GRE sequence (Fig. 12).

Chemical shift artifact

This is an artifact associated with fat that occurs in the frequency-encoded direction of the image because of differences in regional chemical environments surrounding the hydrogen nuclei. This artifact is seen when fat and water are adjacent, and it is caused by differing precessional frequencies of the hydrogen atoms within these tissues. The precessional difference results in misregistration of the proton signals in fat and water, which translates into a dark rim on one edge of an object and a bright rim on the other edge (Fig. 13).

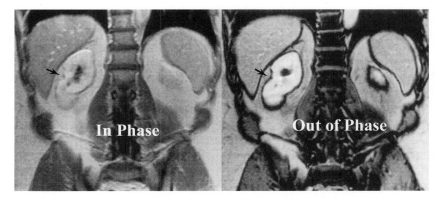

Fig. 12. In-phase and out-of-phase images of the human abdomen. In-phase image is on the left, and out-of-phase image is on the right. The fat around the kidney is nulled on the out-of-phase image because of the adjacent water. Notice how the border of the kidney is highlighted in the out-of-phase image, and the renal infarct is more apparent on this image (*arrow*). (*From* Hood MN, Ho VB, Smirniotopoulos JG, et al. Chemical shift: the artifact and clinical tool revisited. Radiographics 1999;19:357–71; with permission.)

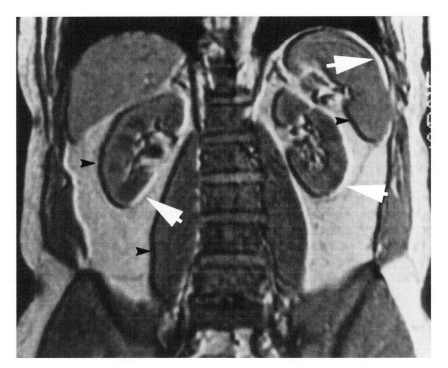

Fig. 13. Chemical shift artifact around the kidneys and musculature in a person caused by fat and water being adjacent. The artifact causes a black edge along one border (*black arrowheads*) of the structure and a white edge on the contralateral border (*white arrowheads*). (*From* Hood MN, Ho VB, Smirniotopoulos JG, et al. Chemical shift: the artifact and clinical tool revisited. Radiographics 1999;19:357–71; with permission.)

Acknowledgment

The author thanks Angela Skidmore for producing several outstanding figures for this article. GE Healthcare General Electric, Milwaukee, Wisconsin; Siemens–Siemens USA, New York, New York; Philips–Philips Medical Systems Bothell, Washington.

References

[1] Bloch F. Nuclear introduction. Physiol Rev 1946;70:460–74.
[2] Available at: http://en.wikipedia.org/wiki/Larmor_precession.
[3] Bloembergen N, Purcell EM, Pound RV. Relaxation effects in nuclear magnetic resonance absorption. Physiol Rev 1948;73:679–712.
[4] Damadian R. Tumor detection by nuclear magnetic resonance. Science 1971;171:1151–3.
[5] Westbrook C, Kaut C. MRI in practice. 2nd edition. Oxford (UK): Blackwell Science; 1998.
[6] Brown MA, Semelka RC. MR imaging abbreviations, definitions, and descriptions: a review. Radiology 1999;213:647–62.

[7] Adair ER, Berglund LG. On the thermoregulatory consequences of NMR imaging. Magn Reson Imaging 1986;4:321–33.

[8] Hahn El. Spin echoes. Physiol Rev 1950;80:580–94.

[9] Meiboom S, Gill D. Modified spin echo method for measuring nuclear relaxation times. Rev Sci Intrum 1958;29:688–91.

[10] Fleckenstein JL, Archer BT, Barker BA, et al. Fast short tau inversion recovery MR imaging. Radiology 1991;179:99–504.

[11] De Doene B, Hajnal JV, Gatehoouse O, et al. MR of the brain using fluid-attenuated inversion recovery (FLAIR) pulse sequences. AJNR Am J Neuroradiol 1992;13:1555–64.

[12] Frahn J, Haase A, Matthaei D. Rapid three-dimensional MR imaging using the FLASH technique. J Comput Assist Tomogr 1986;10:363–8.

[13] Wendt RE 3rd, Wilcott MR 3rd, Nitz W, et al. MR imaging susceptibility-induced magnetic field inhomogeneities. Radiology 1988;168:837–41.

[14] Ogawa S, Lee TM, Kay AR, et al. Brain magnetic resonance imaging with contrast dependent on blood oxygenation. Proc Natl Acad Sci USA 1990;87(24):9868–72.

[15] Hawkes RC, Patz S. Rapid Fourier imaging using steady-state free precession. Magn Reson Med 1987;4:9–23.

[16] Evans AJ, Hedlund LW, Herfkens RJ, et al. Evaluation of steady and pulsatile flow with dynamic MRI using limited flip angles and gradient refocused echoes. Magn Reson Imaging 1987;5:75–482.

[17] Crawley AP, Wood ML, Henkelman RM. Elimination of transverse coherences in FLASH MRI. Magn Reson Med 1988;8:248–60.

[18] Mansfield P. Multiplanar image formation using NMR spin echoes. J Phys C Solid State Phys 1977;10(3):L55–8.

[19] Stejskal EO, Tanner JE. Spin diffusion measurements; spin echoes in the presence of a time-dependent field gradient. J Chem Phys 1965;42:288–92.

[20] Bradley WG Jr, Waluch V, Lai KS, et al. The appearance of rapidly flowing blood on magnetic resonance images. AJR Am J Roentgenol 1984;143:1167–74.

[21] Nishimura DG. Time-of-flight angiography. Magn Reson Med 1990;14:194–201.

[22] Dumoulin CL, Hart HR Jr. Magnetic resonance angiography. Radiology 1986;161:717–20.

[23] Creasy JL, Price RR, Presbrey T, et al. Gadolinium-enhanced MR angiography. Radiology 1990;175:280–3.

[24] Haase A, Frahm J, Hanicke W, et al. 1H NMR chemical shift selective (CHESS) imaging. Phys Med Biol 1985;30:341–4.

[25] Meyer CH, Pauly JM, Macovski A, et al. Simultaneous spatial and spectral selective excitation. Magn Reson Med 1990;15:287–304.

[26] Dixon WT. Simple proton spectroscopic imaging. Radiology 1984;153:189–94.

ELSEVIER
SAUNDERS

Vet Clin Exot Anim 10 (2007) 927–941

VETERINARY
CLINICS
Exotic Animal Practice

Index

Note: Page numbers of article titles are in **boldface** type.

1094-9194/07/$ - see front matter © 2007 Elsevier Inc. All rights reserved.
doi:10.1016/S1094-9194(07)00057-6